"Back in the dawning of the women's conscious raising movement I was amazed to realize I could find out about women's bodies and women's lives directly from other women. Believe me, the idea was revolutionary. Tina Tessina is the nurturing mentor I wish I had at the time. She demonstrates how every woman can find her own best answers. An extremely helpful book."

Isadora Altman
board certified sexologist, LMFT, and author, *Let's Talk Sex, Ask Isadora*

"Dr. Tessina provides a service for women, empowering them to make effective decisions, thereby leveling the playing field with men. A must for the modern woman's reference library."

Richard F. X. O'Connor
Author/editor

"This is a warm and wise book filled with practical advice that applies to women of all ages. Reading it will be one of your best decisions!"

Alison Bell
author and contributing writer to *Complete Woman, Woman's World* and *Parenting*

"This book shows women that they can have it all. Don't let the title fool you, this book is for women of all ages."

The Reverend Dr. Mary Ellen Kilsby

"A highly practical and useful book for anyone who has struggled with making decisions. The information is clear, direct and empowering."
Michelle E. Barone, MA, MFCC
therapist, parent educator and mother

The 10 Smartest Decisions a

WOMAN

Can Make
Before 40

Tina B. Tessina, Ph.D.

Long Beach, CA
United States of America
2nd Edition Copyright 2019 by Tina B. Tessina

Printed in the United States of America by Kindle

For permission, write: tina@tinatessina.com
Muffinhaven Press, Long Beach, CA

Library of Congress Cataloging-in-Publication Data
Tessina, Tina B. The 10 smartest decisions a woman can make before forty Tina B. Tessina. p.213. 2nd Edition ISBN 9781099523458
1. Young women—Life skills guides. 2. Young women—Psychology. 3. Decision making. 4. Self-actualization (Psychology)
1. Title.

10 9 8 7 6 5 4 3 2 1

Original Edition

Copyright © 1998 by Tina Tessina
Published by Health Communications, Inc
Manufactured in the United States of America
2019 edition Cover Design: Panagiotis Lampridis
© 2019 Tina B. Tessina

To young women everywhere who want to create the best life they can. Here's a roadmap to help.

Contents

Acknowledgments

I want to thank: Laurie Harper, my agent, who brought me this idea, and who fought to find a good home for this book.

Christine Belleris and Allison Janse, my editors at HCI who were a big part of its original success. And Panagiotis Lampridis who designed a beautiful new cover.

My secretary, Ronda Oaks, whose organization and helpfulness are invaluable.

My beloved Richard, who always supports me and loves me so very obviously that everyone knows it.

My "friends network" who support me unconditionally: (almost alphabetically) Isadora Alman, Maggie and Eddie Bialack (and their daughter, my goddaughter, Amanda), Victoria Bryan, Ron Creager, David Groves, Sylvia and Glen McWilliams, and Riley Smith.

And I can never forget those who gave me my start: My mom and dad, of course; and my first publishers, Al Saunders and Jeremy Tarcher; Jean Marie Stine, who taught me what editors are all about; and again, Riley K. Smith, who has been the best coauthor anyone could have. These people have made "the impossible dream" easy for me. Many thanks to all of you. You are all blessings in my life, and I love you.

Introduction
Why Women? What Decisions?

***

*Follow your dream . . . take one step
at a time and don't settle for less, just
continue to climb.*

—Amanda Bradley

***

We are in the new millennium—women today are more educated, more well paid and more in control of their lives than their mothers and forebears ever were. Surely these are capable women who know how to make their own decisions. They are single parents, corporate executives or working professionals who are technologically savvy, informed and media aware. Why should they need a book about making decisions?

In years of psychotherapy practice, teaching, leading workshops and lecturing, and watching family and friends, I have seen many people of both genders struggle with decisions. Even the most educated and aware men and women often hesitate when making both long-term and short-term decisions, and many more are very uncomfortable being decisive at all.

Much has been written about the pressures put on men, leading to stress, burnout, heart attacks and other physical and emotional problems. Less is heard about how difficult decision making can be for today's women.

With new technology and conveniences, life is lived at a faster pace than it was for previous generations and it is much more complex than it was for our grandparents, or even our parents.

For example, two generations ago, most women married at a younger age and began the role of stay-at-home mother. Today, cultural expectations and medical advances enable women to have healthy children at a much older age. Therefore, today's women face a myriad of questions: Do I wait to have children and focus on my career? If I do have children, do I choose daycare or do I quit my job to care for them?

More equality exists within marriages today so that decisions concerning child rearing, education and finances require input from both husbands and wives. "How much discipline is necessary?" "How do we protect our children from violence and adult information on television, in movies and on the Internet?" Single women without children also face choices most of our grandmothers and mothers didn't face. "Do I stay at a comfortable yet boring job that pays my bills or do I take a chance and start my own business?"

Many of these decisions would have been incomprehensible thirty years ago, and in every aspect of our lives (home, work, family, friends, entertainment, school) we face the same sort of necessary decisions.

The freedom that we enjoy, compared to women of the past, has also left us with much more decision-making responsibility. The many women who attend my lectures and workshops and those who are clients in my private practice repeatedly express how stressed they are by the decisions they must make.

More control, and therefore more responsibility, is in women's hands today than ever before, and no matter how competent and well-educated, no matter how successful a woman is, she may not feel secure that she knows the right decisions for herself. Many women hesitate to make a decision because they don't want to make a mistake, and with good reason.

Young women, just starting out on a career with little life experience beyond schooling, can feel pressured by expectations that they should be "Superwomen" ready to take on the world. They feel they must be computer and Internet savvy, competent in their new career and self-assured in all their decisions.

In our more individual-focused society, a woman may be raising her family as a single parent; she may be isolated in a business career still mostly dominated by men; or she may have moved halfway across the country, miles from family and childhood friendships. Such women are separated from the old-style extended family support networks that used to give advice and feedback.

In addition, today's technology changes so fast, and expectations and mores are so different from previous generations, that feedback, if we receive it, may be virtually meaningless in the context of our postmodern lives.

For example, women with careers may not be able to get the kind of advice they need from their mothers, aunts and other older women who may not have worked. Men who have had careers may offer advice that misses the point because it comes from their male experience and does not account for the importance a woman may place on family, relationships or security. Women from lower socioeconomic levels who work very hard to get a college education may receive hostile responses from family and childhood friends, such as, "You think you're so much better than we are."

Often women don't make more effective decisions because they don't realize they have to! Young women who are overwhelmed by the numerous daily decisions they have to make can easily forget to plan for the future. Raised by families whose expectations for girls may be old-fashioned, and in an educational system whose methods may lag behind the demands of society, young women are often not given the skills they need to be decisive and plan ahead. Instead women often drift along until a crisis occurs, at which time it's often too late to do anything but solve problems.

You don't have to fall into this trap. Intuitive hunches are not sufficient for organizing a demanding life. Guesses are not good enough to determine where you'll live, whether you'll work or not, and what your standard of living will be. This problem often does not appear significant until age thirty. At that point, however, you may begin to suspect you haven't made enough conscious and effective decisions to maximize your life opportunities.

CULTURAL BIAS

If you feel confused or unsure about the decisions you have made or need to make, you are not alone. Women often have not been praised for using the power of decision making; in fact, when women such as Oprah Winfrey, Barbra Streisand or Secretary of State and Presidential candidate Hillary Clinton stretch beyond their "acceptable" roles and make smart business or political decisions, they are often criticized. The message? Women who "overstep" their bounds are disagreeable and shrewish. Whether you are aware of it or not, this bias may make you reluctant to be decisive and can hamper your learning how to make decisions effectively.

This attitude and cultural bias can keep you stuck in three ways:

1. *Lack of decision-making expertise.* Confidence comes with knowledge and experience, and if you have been discouraged from making decisions on your own, when you need to make an important or sudden decision you may feel completely unprepared. If you lack an adequate support system of wise friends or family members who can discuss problems and issues with you, it is much more difficult to feel secure in your own mind. If you believe women are not supposed to be decisive and rational thinkers,

you may lack the information you need to make good decisions, including information about yourself. While it can be helpful if you have learned to see yourself and your life in emotional and intuitive terms, it is not sufficient to replace effective decision making.

Women with this outlook often display distaste at the idea of having good judgment and intellectual clarity, dismissing it as "cold" and "unfeeling." Without the ability to see yourself unemotionally and rationally, you won't accurately see or acknowledge your real limits and strengths, and you'll have trouble distinguishing the difference between reality and your wishes. To the extent that this is your problem, the decisions you make will be unsuited or unrealistic for your abilities and can set you up for failure. If you don't understand from experience that decision making includes experimentation and learning from mistakes, you'll become discouraged and more convinced that decision making is not for you.

2. *Making feelings more important than decisions.* Today's society is the beneficiary of 100 years of psychotherapy. Its influence has encouraged contemporary women to place a high value upon emotional understanding, open communication and getting in touch with our feelings. Unfortunately, placing too much emphasis on

how we feel can get in the way of making clear-cut decisions. It's possible to get stuck in helplessness, encouraged by the current climate of victimization, which seems to maintain that you can't move forward until you work through years of "recovery." Even in therapy, the therapist may focus so much on your feelings that you don't learn the necessary skills to be decisive. Of course your feelings are important, and I would never recommend that you ignore them, but the ability to put feelings aside, think clearly and rationally, and often even go against what feels good is essential to making sound decisions. Men have often been criticized for being too unemotional and logical, but they are usually considered capable of making good decisions. It is both possible and desirable to create a balance between emotional reaction and responses and rational, objective decision making.

3. *Being intuitive, not decisive.* Even in today's supposedly enlightened atmosphere, women are still considered the keepers of warmth and connectedness in the culture. We are encouraged to honor our feelings and other right-brain, intuitive and emotional processes but not to balance it with solid, left-brain, rational thinking processes. While intuition and spiritual philosophy can be very enjoyable and lend

deeper meaning to your life, they are not very compatible with the concrete decision-making skills and practical thinking you need to make thought-out, rational and farseeing decisions. All great thinkers have hunches and flashes of insight, but great decisions are made only when those hunches are checked for accuracy. You need self-empowering, reality-based ideas to make the decisions necessary to take responsibility for yourself, and to develop self-control.

"Our passions, when well exercised, have wisdom; they guide our thinking, our values, our survival," writes Dr. Daniel Goleman in his bestseller, *Emotional Intelligence.* "But they can easily go awry, and do so all too often." It is very possible, and highly desirable, to be decisive as well as intuitive, rational as well as emotionally aware. The woman who learns to develop these skills has gained a priceless tool for creating a successful life. As most women have spent most of their lives developing their emotional side, it is time to focus on the rational: the ability to decide.

HOW TO BENEFIT FROM THE EXPERIENCE OF OTHER WOMEN

Although the quality of your later years will depend largely on the decisions you make today, you don't have to reinvent the wheel. The experience of other women, who blazed many of the same trails you will travel, can be very useful. This book is an opportunity to look into other women's lives to see the decisions they made before forty— good and bad—and the results. Out of their personal experiences comes "The 10 Smartest Decisions" you can make to create a life for yourself that is full of loving and supportive affiliations and a reliable road to financial security, whatever your background, education or history.

THE TOP 10: GOOD DECISIONS AND THE POWER TO MAKE THEM

Look around you. Some of your friends and colleagues are living happy lives, with relative financial security, good relationships and friendships, and promising futures. They appear contented with their lives, for the most part. Others seem to flounder. They're long on dreams but short on practicality. They may be overwhelmed by too many demands at once, thus emotionally and physically falling apart. Their goals may be interesting but are either unsuited to their real capacities or unlikely to lead to long-term financial or emotional security.

Is the discrepancy between success and floundering only an accident? Does one group really start off with more advantages than the other? Are those who do well in life luckier than those who do poorly? If you look into these women's lives, you'll find that some of those with the worst beginnings are doing best, and some of those with the "luckiest" origins are floundering.

What makes the difference? Why are some women apparently living the life they want, despite whatever adversity life has given them, while others seem to make mistake after mistake, no matter how hard they try? More important, what will the next few decades of your own life be like? Do you know what you want and how to get it?

Women today have more freedom, opportunity and responsibility than ever before. You are more likely to have a career, be a single parent, and be geographically separated from your family and childhood friends. Therefore, along with the freedom, you may also feel more isolated, overwhelmed and alienated than ever before. As a generation, women today are more educated, technically savvy, and politically aware and, as a consequence, they feel more career pressures and anxieties. Today you have the power to make your own decisions, and you probably feel more anxiety about it. The sword of freedom cuts both ways: Educated women are becoming everything from medical doctors to politicians to astronauts, while young and disadvantaged women are left on their own without support. Three generations ago, a decisive woman was rare, an oddity. Today, the quality of your life often depends solely on the caliber of your decision-making skills.

As a long-time therapist, I've watched many women between eighteen and forty struggle to learn the skills today's life requires, and I've seen the results of both wonderful and terrible decisions they have made. In that time, I've learned that, while luck or circumstances, good and bad, will play a part in your life, it is your *reaction* and *response* to your circumstances and how well you make *decisions* that will be the real determining factors in your subsequent happiness.

More important than a happy or affluent childhood (who hasn't seen children of the rich and famous with completely messed-up lives?) and more important than luck (we have all seen people fail to take advantage of lucky breaks) is the ability to make effective and realistic decisions. Even with the best advantages and education, you can feel out of control and miserable with your life, while with the right decisions you can surmount enormous obstacles and wind up thriving, emotionally and physically.

WOMEN'S STORIES

In this book, we will examine the stories of several women, ages twenty-five to thirty-nine, and the decisions they face:

Jodie, thirty-six, was in Junior Achievers in high school and got lucky. Her business, a restaurant-to-home delivery service, became successful, and Jodie became one of the country's youngest entrepreneurs. However, the excitement of business success has worn off, and managing employees and finances has become hard work. "When will life get to be fun again?" Jodie wonders. "I have no time for friends or fun. All my friends went to college and are having a great time now. Sure, they studied hard, and after graduation they all got jobs, but not one of them works the long hours I do. Being self-employed means never having a day off, no vacations, no holidays, no weekends. Business problems are always coming up. I've loved being successful, and I've even gotten a little famous, which is fun, but it doesn't replace having a real life." What decisions does she need to make to put her life back in order?

Kim, twenty-four, has followed the strict rules of her immigrant family all her life. Those strong family guidelines helped her succeed and finish college with a pre-med degree. Now she is having doubts that what her family wants for her is what she really wants. She faces many more grueling years of medical school if she follows their wishes, and she's afraid she'll wind up unhappy and stuck in a very demanding career she doesn't like. "My family really sacrificed for me, and I love them. I want them to be proud, and I have a debt to repay them. I'm very grateful for their love and support. But I worry that being a medical doctor will be too tough for me. It's a big step, and I'm not sure it's the right one. What if I get into medical school and I can't make it? What if I don't like medicine enough to spend my life as a doctor? What kinds of medical careers are available to me? My family is sweet and loving and very old-fashioned. They don't know any more about what it takes to become a doctor than I do. How can I disappoint them? I can't even tell them about my doubts, because they wouldn't understand. I just don't know what to do." How can Kim decide to think for herself and make her own decisions?

Kisha, twenty-six, was a rebellious teenager from an economically deprived background. She became a single mother at sixteen and gave birth again at eighteen but then changed her priorities, took advantage of some programs for welfare moms, and got herself through a trade school and off welfare. She now has a certificate in computer science and a pretty good job. She's proud of her accomplishments but still not sure what decisions are right for herself and her children. She's struggling to hold a job, take care of her family, and build a life for them all, and she can see the world of computers moving so fast she's not sure she can keep up. "I'm proud of myself," says Kisha. "I've come a long way from how I grew up. But it seems the more I learn, the more I realize what I don't know. I was brought up with a lot of love but not encouraged to stay in school or to learn new things. I don't want to bring my children up the same way—I want them to want to learn and grow, but how do I guide them? Sometimes I feel so alone in the world, as though I'm the only mom who ever had these problems. And I have trouble knowing I'm making the right career decisions. Who can I turn to? Who can I ask for advice?" What help can Kisha get in making the decisions she needs to keep her life going in the right direction?

Marie, thirty-one, is in love with music, particularly opera. After getting a degree in music education, she briefly tried a professional singing career but decided that it took the fun out of music for her. She teaches music in high school and has summers off. She wants to travel to hear and see her favorite operas and singers in the famous houses of Europe, but she worries that her life is too focused on her hobby and that in later years she'll regret not settling down and raising a family. "I love my life now, and teaching high school students to love music is very rewarding. I can't imagine life without my love of opera and traveling in Europe to hear the great performers in the great opera houses—the Paris Opera, La Scala, the music festivals—it's my greatest thrill. I'd love to meet someone who shares my passion for opera, but I don't know if I'd ever want a family. Everyone tells me I'll regret it if I don't, but the women I know who have grown children seem to have lots of problems. What if teaching other people's children turns out not to be enough?" How can Marie decide what will satisfy her in the future?

Megan, thirty-four, always wanted children but, being a bright student, she postponed thinking about marriage and family to get her law degree. Now she works for a large law partnership, which is encouraging her to get on the "partner track," but Megan knows that means "living" her job and dedicating the better portion of her life to it, and she still worries about eventually having children. "Most of the young lawyers in my company would give anything to be getting all the encouragement I'm getting—but there's another side to it. I know that the partners expect up-and-coming lawyers to put in extra hours and to make the law firm their whole life. That would be okay for now, but I don't know whether I could ever find the time to be married, much less to be a good mom. As a partner in this prestigious law firm, I know I'll have a lot of money, and many opportunities—but can I take the chance that I'll never have the marriage and family I long for?" How does she decide whether the mommy track or the partner track is right for her?

Rita, thirty-one, got married right out of high school and had two children. Her husband, Ron, has a successful business as an insurance agent, but when the children were old enough to go to school, Rita decided to go to work, partly because she wanted the stimulation and partly to make extra money so the children could go to private school. Now she feels stressed, overwhelmed and worried that she's not a good enough mother. "I know a lot of women who think I have the ideal life, and in a lot of ways I do," Rita explains. "Ron is a good man, and we have a good marriage and a lovely family life. I feel guilty when I think that should be enough for me. But as soon as the children were in preschool, I was really bored at home—I wasn't using my mind enough. I wasn't stimulated. Work is fun for me, most of the time. I love being with other people, getting recognition for my efforts, and the extra money doesn't hurt, either. But I hear that being with your children all the time is important. I'm a lot happier, even though I get overloaded sometimes. Still, I wonder if my children are paying a price for my happiness. Am I doing the right thing?" How does she decide what her priorities should be?

Robin, thirty-seven, always dreamed of being a counselor, and she finally went back to school and earned her associate's degree and license in alcoholism counseling. She has tried working in counseling centers, but she really wants to work for herself. She feels that college taught her nothing about the business of counseling or about starting a practice. "I feel as if I know a lot about counseling and alcoholism—some of it I learned in my own family. I'm an expert there. But no one said a word during my education about how to begin a business. I haven't a clue how to start my own practice, and I don't really want to work for anyone else. I have some great ideas about starting a treatment center, but where do I begin?" How can Robin find out what she needs to know?

Sharon, twenty-five, was fortunate enough to have her parents put her through a good college, where she got her MBA. Now the job offers are not as good as she hoped, and she faces having to move to another city to get a good job or taking a lesser position so she can stay in the city where her friends and family are. "Home is very important to me, and I'm very close to my family and friends. I want to have a successful career, and I feel lucky to have gone to college, but in this small town

I can't get a really good position. My classmates are all moving to big cities where the big careers are, but I don't think I'd like living too far away. Is it wrong for me to want to stay at home? I'm afraid whatever decision I make will ruin the rest of my life. I'm very torn." How does she decide between a career and living where she's comfortable?

These women all face decisions, and the results of prior decisions, that will affect their success and happiness for years to come. These decisions can be life-changing. We will follow their stories throughout the book, and watch what happens as they face the most important decisions so far in their lives.

There are many decisions that once made are not easy to correct. The good news is that, like these young women, anyone can learn effective decision making. This book will show you how.

WHAT THIS BOOK IS ABOUT

This is not an ordinary women's book about meeting and marrying a great guy, solving your sex problems or raising kids successfully. It is not about getting everything you want in life, and it's certainly not about avoiding failure, or feeling like a failure. No. It's much more realistic than that.

In this book, you will see how making a few good decisions before you're forty is likely to provide you with a *real* life of relative comfort, security, fun, and affection, as well as enough flexibility to adapt to fluctuating life circumstances— such as changing economic conditions, your own attitudes changing as you mature and new life circumstances. Wanting success means facing failure; no one who succeeds does so without failing many times. By making the correct decisions now, you can prepare yourself to land on your feet after a failure and to cope effectively with the good and bad surprises life is bound to bring. Your ability to do so is always dependent on how well you make decisions, and the decisions you make by age forty can make your early years more productive—and the later years much easier.

You can let your life lead you until you feel completely hopeless and helpless, or you can respond, even to difficult circumstances, by making good decisions that lead you to satisfaction and security. If you are fortunate enough to understand the process and principles of making good decisions, you can, despite setbacks, obstacles and changes, build a life for yourself that you will enjoy. Valuable ideas and the steps you need to follow to make good decisions are presented in chapter 1, "The Power of a Good Decision."

PERFECTION IS NOT NECESSARY

Some of the women you just read about had trouble making any decision because they were afraid of making the wrong one and because they thought they should be able to read the future and know that whatever they decide *must* work out for a lifetime. Focusing too much on what can go wrong led them, and could lead you, to paralysis. Of course no decision will be perfect, and things will go wrong; the many unpredictable twists and turns of life make it impossible to prepare in advance for them all. But, as you will see in chapter 1, part of the decision-making process is learning how to tell when a decision needs to be reevaluated. Each of these women learned to make the decisions that made their lives work—and so can you.

These 10 Smartest Decisions have worked well for many women, and the practice of evaluating and experimenting with them will give you the experience you need to become an effective decision maker. In the following chapters, you will become familiar with all of the decisions, learn the skills involved in implementing them and see how other women, like you, have used them.

THE 10 SMARTEST DECISIONS A WOMAN CAN MAKE BEFORE 40

1. Decide to Make Intelligent Choices

2. Decide to Resolve Old Issues

3. Decide to Set Realistic Goals and Priorities

4. Decide to Make the Most of Who You Are

5. Decide to Get the Education and Training You Need

6. Decide to Be an Effective Communicator

7. Decide to Keep Learning

8. Decide to Build Personal and Professional Networks

9. Decide to Create Financial Security

10. Decide to Balance Work and Play

This book offers practical advice about why these decisions are so important, why they work and how to make them, taking into account the realities of today's economy and shifting employment scene and that any woman who wants to improve her life can. Each chapter focuses on one area requiring a decision, using examples from the lives of the young women mentioned earlier. You will read about how making, or not making, various decisions affected them; how they approached their decisions; and what they ultimately decided to do. You will also learn why each decision is so crucial to a successful life; and you will find information and simple steps to help you adapt the decision to your own life circumstances. By implementing these decisions, you can build a life of loving and supportive affiliations, the "support network" that is so vital to good mental and physical health. These decisions will also help you discover a simple and effective road to financial security, even in an unpredictable economy. You will learn to set and follow priorities, choose the path that is right for you, and acquire the training, education, and information you need to fulfill your promise.

While some of these decisions seem simple, obvious and self-explanatory to the women who already use them, others are revelations; whether they are obvious or life altering varies greatly from woman to woman. Even if you feel comfortable that you understand all the decisions, you'll find that the information and examples provided will actually help you implement these decisions in your life.

I offer this book in the spirit of sharing the experience that years of working and living have taught me. Here is the information that years of counseling have taught me most women need. As you learn to make and implement these decisions, I know you will soon see the benefits and results in your own life.

This book presents the decisions clearly and concisely, paying you the compliment of assuming that, if you are intelligent and assertive enough to buy and read a self-help book, you can implement the suggestions within it. It does not take the attitude that you will *of course* do what it recommends but rather presents an intelligent and well-developed argument, based on experience and illustrated by women's stories, for why it works.

IF YOU'RE OVER 40

In speaking to women about this book as I wrote it, the most frequent comment I heard from women forty and over was: "It's too late for me." No, it's not too late. These decisions will work for anyone at any age. Although the suggested optimum time of life to make these decisions is before age forty, it is never too late to implement them, so if you are forty or over you need not be discouraged. You can improve your life at any age with *The 10 Smartest Decisions a Woman Can Make Before 40*.

And now, you can get *The 10 Smartest Decisions a Woman Can Make After Forty*

https://tinyurl.com/yctuql47

1

The Power of a Good Decision: Decide to Make Intelligent Choices

You don't get to choose how you're going to die. Or when. You can only decide how you're going to live. Now.

—Joan Baez

Smart decisions are not accidental. They are based on five basic aspects: self-awareness, research, appropriateness, support and self-respect. Knowing these aspects, making sure your decisions are based on them, and understanding how to use them will help you distinguish a good decision from a poor one.

YOUR KEY TO GOOD DECISIONS

The secret that enables you as a woman to be decisive— that is, to make a decision, to trust that decision and to carry it out—is that you know your decisions are sound because they're based on sound principles. Since, as women, we have often been rewarded more for being decorative or supportive than we have for being decisive, we may not always feel secure in our decision-making skills. Researchers in schools have long observed that boys tend to be more independent and competitive, while girls tend to be more cooperative and to want to be supported and to belong. In short, boys work more individually, making up their own minds, while girls tend to work in groups, cooperating and looking for consensus. Many argue about whether these traits are genetically based or socially bred, but few people disagree that they exist.

FIVE BASIC ASPECTS OF A GOOD DECISION

One of the benefits of learning the five basic aspects of good decisions, in addition to the results of the decisions themselves, is that while you're learning you're also developing abilities and enhancing your self-respect. If making decisions or knowing which decisions are right for you is difficult, in the struggle to learn you are also building your self-esteem.

Aspect 1: Self-Awareness

All good decisions must be based on self-knowledge as well as knowledge of the facts and circumstances. Who you are will perhaps affect the outcome of your decisions more than any other factor. The same decision that might be good for someone else might be bad for you.

There are many ways you know yourself. For example, you know many of your likes and dislikes, how comfortable or uncomfortable you feel in certain situations, and whether you're an introvert or an extrovert. Most of us have been distracted from paying attention to ourselves because we are busy, stressed or focused on someone else. However, it is often the unknown aspects of our personalities that help us make sound decisions—or prevent us from making them.

Hidden anger, for example, can keep you from looking at the facts related to the anger, so you cannot make accurate judgments based on whole facts.

***Rita** has a lot of anger toward her husband, Ron, because he resisted the changes she wanted to make when she went back to work, and consequently she didn't evaluate her decision clearly or talk it over thoroughly with him. To overcome her anxiety, she took the first opportunity that presented itself, and now she's not sure she made the right decision. Her anger at Ron, added to her fear of making the change, prevented her from taking the time she needed to think things through. Now she realizes that not taking enough time to get the facts was a mistake. Ron's resistance to the changes her job made in their family life made Rita anxious, and her anxiety affected her ability to take the time she needed to do research. She might, for example, have worked as a temporary worker for a while to see what different types of jobs were like and to acquire firsthand experience of how working would affect her time with her family.*

Rita's most recent job experience taught her a lot about herself. She now realizes how much she loves being responsible for her job and appreciated for it, how much she likes interacting with her coworkers, and also how much her family means to her. She is much more torn by these conflicting issues than she realized she would be. "I love working, and I love my family. It came as a complete surprise how much different the reality is from my original idea. It's very important to me to be recognized for my accomplishments beyond being a wife and mother. As a career woman, I feel like an individual, making my own decisions and even my own mistakes, and getting direct results. As a wife and mother, I love being the one who makes the family run smoothly, and I feel very close to my husband and children. It's as if there are two different parts of me that crave recognition—one wants to belong to others, one wants to be acknowledged as an individual. Sometimes the two parts of me struggle with each other."

Knowing as much as you can about what you want, what your weaknesses and strong points and talents and abilities are, and checking all your decisions to see if they're appropriate for you will help you make decisions you can live with happily.

KEEP A JOURNAL

To know yourself better, I recommend keeping a diary or journal about your feelings and reactions to your life. You can use the diary as a place to look at yourself and your life as though you are watching a character in a movie and evaluating that character's (your) strengths and weaknesses. You can also ask friends and family members for their observations about your personality traits and attributes. Choose supportive people; you don't want to glean a lot of critical comments, just honest and kind observations.

*When **Megan** was confused about whether to have children or pursue her legal career, she asked her friends for their input. Most told her she was wonderful with other people's children and seemed a lot happier around them, so perhaps she should consider the mommy track or some other way to combine motherhood and a career. Some members of her family, however, told her that she had always wanted to have a career, and being an attorney seemed to suit her personality, so they didn't think she should give up her career entirely. Megan began to write her thoughts and feelings about her career in a journal, making notes about all the reactions she got from family and friends, and arguing with these comments privately in her writings. She wrote out all her feelings, pro and con, and as she wrote she began to see her thoughts more clearly, understanding them better because she could analyze them in written form. Taking the time to write, which was a very private and safe form of "thinking out loud," calmed her and gave her a chance to think more clearly.*

"For a while, there seemed to be constant static in my mind—ideas would swirl around, gone before I could really find out what they were," says Megan. "Writing my thoughts in my journal helped me to slow down and really understand what I was thinking. It was a shock to find out how much I argued with myself over everything. There was my opinion of what I should do, then there was my idea of what everyone else thought I should do, and then there was what others actually told me I should do. It was all very confusing. Writing it down helped me sort out what I really thought, and it also quieted my internal chaos. It was a surprise to me to realize that all my ideas did not necessarily have to be in conflict. I discovered I could have my cake and eat it, too." Eventually, Megan decided both viewpoints were accurate and that finding a way to be both a mother and a lawyer was what would make her happy. She decided to focus on family law and custody cases and to work part-time if she ever became pregnant.

Sometimes the decision you need to make is very close to what you are doing, but somehow it feels wrong or out of focus. This can happen because you are being "helped" too much or too stridently by others. When others want what they think is best for you, and you care for them, it can be difficult to know your own mind.

*Because of her respect and reverence for her family and for tradition, **Kim** has done all the work to earn a pre-med degree, which her* *parents wanted, but now that she faces years of difficult training and education to become an M.D., she wonders if medicine is truly the right career for her. She decided to go to therapy and sort through her feelings before making her decision. Almost immediately, her therapist began to focus on Kim's own opinions about what she was doing, and for the first time Kim learned to evaluate her own opinions, rather than considering only what others thought.*

"I came to realize, with my therapist's help, that I never recognized myself as a grown-up person, or allowed myself to be in charge of my own life," says Kim now. "Once I learned to value my own opinion, and to give myself credit for being able to make good decisions, I was able to put everyone else's advice into perspective. I can learn from others now, but I don't have to let them make my decisions for me." Learning more self-awareness was a real eye-opener for Kim. She became aware of how much she wanted to do good in the world and how important it was to her personally to help people. She decided that surgery or emergency medicine would be too difficult and unpleasant for her, but she enjoys children and families, so Kim is now happily embarked on her medical training and planning to be a pediatrician with a family practice in the town where she lives. She wants to focus more on preventive medicine and early childhood care than on serious diseases or surgical procedures. Now she feels sure that this decision is hers, and

she has the added joy that it makes her family happy, too.

As with Kim, the right decision for you may be obscured by the wishes of your parents, spouse, best friend or coworker. Caring about these people, not wanting to make waves, or just not wanting to deal with their disappointment or criticism can make it difficult to think clearly and to know what you want. If Kim had either rebelled or complied with her family's wishes, she would have made the wrong decision. She needed to find out what *she* wanted, whether or not it was in line with what her family wanted.

PLAN A AND PLAN B

Sometimes the solution lies in preparing for more than one decision simultaneously—as in having a Plan A and a Plan B. This is especially useful if your original plan involves a lot of unknowns or risks.

Marie, the gifted singer, knows enough about herself to follow her passion, but she is not certain that passion will last. There are also many unknowns about how successful she could be in a singing career. Careers in the arts are notoriously difficult. "I know myself well enough to know I don't do well under too much pressure," explains Marie. "Having the expectations and stresses of a singing career might take all the joy out of it for me. I also love inspiring others with what I know, and teaching young people to appreciate the magic of music is thrilling to me. If I got the opportunity again for a singing career, I would certainly try it, but I'd better have something to fall back on." Marie decided her Plan B would be to get a teaching credential, which provides a secure and rewarding career for her; it also allows her to indulge her passion for music now and provides a solid base for changes in the future.

Accept the Facts

Often, the key to a solution eludes you because you haven't looked at the simple surface aspects of the situation.

"I worked so hard on my education," says **Sharon**, *"and the reward was supposed to be an excellent position with a good salary. But as I began looking, I was terribly disappointed to find out all the best jobs were in the big cities, and not close to home. I don't think I'll find a really good position in my small city—but I want to live here, not in some big, strange place. I really need to refocus on what is more important to me."* Taking the time to see that she loves the climate, her friends and family, and the cozy familiarity of where she lives now, and momentarily changing her focus from *"career prestige,"* allows her to see that a job away from home, no matter how good, will probably make her unhappy in the long run. Staying where the sun shines more often, as well as where her close family and friends are, may make the difference between having the energy to

succeed (even if she has to start from a lower position) and being too overwhelmed to try.

Self-awareness gives you the ability and will to face your limitations as well as your strengths and accept them, which can sometimes be painful.

Jodie, the entrepreneur, built her home delivery service, Dinners to You, from scratch and loves it like a child, but she is completely overwhelmed by its success. Selling it, or expanding and going public, which means letting someone else control it, might be painful for her, but it also might allow her to move on to new things that work much better for her. "It's so hard to give up control of the business," Jodie explains. "I've had full control over it from the beginning—it was my idea, and everything was done my way. But now, it feels as though it's controlling me. I had to realize that the business had grown so much I couldn't take care of it all by myself any more. I hate to admit it, but it's not fun anymore, and I'm over my head. I never thought the business would grow so much I couldn't handle it. I was just caught up in the excitement. But now I'm getting burned out, and even making bad decisions. I guess it's time to admit that I need some help, and to get it I suppose I have to give up some of the control."

Self-awareness is indeed fundamental to making good decisions, as these women's experiences show. In chapter 4, "Who Loves Ya, Baby?" we'll explore in more detail how these women used this principle to make great decisions, and also how you can do the same.

Aspect 2: Research

Good decisions are the result of a great deal of research. Although a hunch, intuition, or your astrological chart may provide inspiration and creative ideas, those ideas will not become reality until you make sure you get the appropriate facts. There is no substitute for solid information to help you decide. There are many sources of information all around you. Libraries, others who have more experience in the area, the Internet, books, and a thoughtful review of your own and others' past experiences are all good sources of data. In fact, for clients who feel stuck and can't decide something, I often suggest research, and I find that people are often indecisive because they actually don't have enough information to make a good decision. If you feel hesitant about making a decision, perhaps you are trying to make it based on guesswork and intuition, instead of solid information.

For example, if you're a career woman, like Megan the attorney, and considering having a baby, you can read in books and online magazines about the joys and complications of being a working mom, talk to other working moms, and find out what the rules are in your company and other places where you can work. With enough information in advance, you can set things up creatively to accommodate both motherhood and your career. Perhaps you, like many others today, can find a way to work at home more via computer and phone and spend less time at the office. If you look in magazines or on the Internet, you can find local classes, books and articles that will give you plenty of related information. Don't fall into the trap of thinking what you want to do is impossible before you've thoroughly researched it. You may find, as Megan did, that you can have your dream and live it, too.

To research a big decision, such as a change in your career, it's worth spending a few months doing informational interviews with those working in the field, volunteering in a related area to find out if you like it, taking classes in that subject—anything to get more information and experience before you actually make a decision that will affect you for years to come.

When a good job offer in another state came through for **Sharon**, *she did a lot of research and thoroughly checked out the area to which she might be moving. She wanted to know about the prices, the social life, the year-round weather, the school systems for her (future) children and, most of all, about leaving everything familiar. In Sharon's case, doing the research was part of what convinced her it would be very difficult to begin life anew in an unfamiliar location. "The more I traveled and looked at other places, and the more I imagined what life would be like away from my hometown, the more unhappy I became," she says. "It was a very good job, and if it were here I would be happy to have it—but the price, moving away from everything and everyone I love, was way too high. Getting an actual offer really brought everything into sharp focus for me. I realized that I could begin lower,* *at one of the jobs available here, even though it had much less prestige and a smaller salary, and with a few years of dedication I could work my way up to almost the same level. It would be a slower start, but I would be where I want to be, and I wouldn't have to begin the rest of my life all over again. Prestige is just not as important to me as the people and the home I love so much. If I hadn't tried looking in the other places and hadn't gone to the job interviews, I never would have known which was more important to me."*

Moving to a new state, city or country after just a few visits or vacations in the area amounts to making a very big commitment without enough research. Thorough research about the area, including getting yourself established in some social networks *before* you make the move will give you enough information to make an informed decision. In chapter 8, "It Takes a Village," we'll see how women have done this.

Proper research can save you lots of disappointment, so make certain that your decisions are based in reality and have a high chance of being successful.

The Components of Research

The major components of research are: (1) your own experience, (2) the experience of others you know and (3) the available information. Using all three of these components means you will have enough information to make an informed decision.

Your Own Experience

There is no better research than what you have seen with your own eyes, heard with your own ears, and learned from your own experience, but this information will do you no good if you don't use it. It's often easy, in the stress and excitement of a new choice, to forget to think about your prior experience. Whenever you're considering a decision, make sure you consciously review your experiences that relate to that decision. **Sharon**, for example, drew on her own experience of how important her surroundings were to her and how uncomfortable she was in strange places to support her decision to stay in her hometown.

To draw on your own experience, it's often helpful to make a list of what you know about the subject, time, place or persons involved in your decision. Over a period of several days, add to your list, divide it into pros and cons and talk to trusted friends about what your past experiences have been.

The Experience of Others

Contemplating doing something you have never done can be pretty scary. Being the first in your family, or the first woman in your family, to go to college, to move to another area, to take an executive position or to move to another country is like stepping off a cliff into the unknown. Contemplating it can be scary enough to leave you feeling paralyzed.

When my first book was completed in 1980, I did not know anyone who had written a book or had done a promotional tour or TV or radio interviews, and my reaction was panic. The publicist hired by my publisher taught me how to interview, taped mock TV and radio interviews, and made sure I had a chance to talk to other authors.

Once I acquired the benefits of the very supportive publicist's experience, and that of other authors, I was able to calm down and get through the first few interviews, after which I felt more at ease. To this day, I find it helpful to talk to other authors, and I belong to an organization called the American Society of Journalists and Authors (www.ASJA.org), so I can share experiences with others in the same field. Now, many years and books later, I also have friends who are authors with whom I can share experiences and information.

No matter what experience you're facing: marriage, college, mountain climbing, a new place to live, entering politics, or having a child; you can learn a lot by talking to people who've been there and done it themselves. If you don't know anyone with that experience, you can find an expert in the following ways:

1. Ask people you know to introduce you to someone with that experience.

2. Attend a class, a lecture or a book signing by an expert in the field.

3. Read a biography or first-person account.

4. Research and ask questions online.

5. Call a college or business with experts in that topic and ask to speak to an expert.

6. Go to a meeting of a group or organization in that field.

7. Search the archives of your local newspaper for a related story and call the reporter or the people mentioned in the story.

Available Information

If you don't get all the information you need from your own experience or that of others, there's always information available in the library, on the Internet or through nonprofit organizations. It's always valuable to patronize your local library and get to know your librarian. Libraries are part of a national and international network of information, and a good librarian can help you find information from all over the world. Libraries have archives of years' worth of newspapers and magazines, and they often have video, audio, and Internet access. Librarians can also help you find pertinent local and national organizations whose staff often know what is going on in related subjects. Even if you could find the same information online, the help of an experienced librarian can be invaluable.

Your very knowledgeable and helpful local librarian can even help you find information that the library doesn't carry, through reference books that list special organizations, museums, archives and private specialty libraries. If there is a local university, college or community college in your area, its library can be equally helpful, especially in the areas in which the school grants diplomas.

Aspect 3: Appropriateness

A good decision is appropriate to you, your life circumstances, your goals and your other decisions. For example, when **Rita**'s children were very young, she felt it was inappropriate for her to consider a career. However, now that they are in school, she has an opportunity to make a big change: to get training or education that would allow her to work in a way that's compatible with raising her family. The same decision that would have been inappropriate two years ago is very fitting now. "I would have been very unhappy being away from my children when they were small." Rita smiles at the memory. "And I know I'm lucky to have had the choice. But when they began school, they didn't need me as much, and I needed more challenge. It was the perfect time for me to try something new."

Your decisions often affect others in your life, too. Not only do good decisions need to fit in with the aspects of your own personality or life; they also must be appropriate to the others who may be affected.

Kim wants to honor her very traditional family but must also make sure her life-shaping decisions suit her by considering the appropriateness of going to medical school. Rather than just giving in to family pressure, she is more likely to make a decision that will make her happy. "After I realized how pressured and unhappy I felt, and I figured out what I wanted, I explained it to my family," Kim says, "and they were more understanding than I realized. They just wanted me to be happy and successful, and they thought medical school was right for me. I know now that they would have been very

*unhappy if I had let myself go on being miserable.
I realize that by taking the time to figure out what
I wanted, we all had a better chance to be
satisfied."*

To make sure your decision will be appropriate, it is necessary to analyze how it will affect your life and the life of those you care about. The appropriateness of your decision will affect how well you can maintain and follow through on it. If Kim had tried to do what her family wanted without making sure it was appropriate for her, odds are that she wouldn't have had the motivation and dedication she needed to accomplish something as difficult as completing her M.D.

A decision that's appropriate for you is a decision you have considered and evaluated carefully, in advance, and for which you have anticipated the effect it will have on your life. A decision that suits your character, your ethics, your personality and your style will be much more effective because it will be much easier to carry out. Self-awareness is crucial to making this comparison, and being proactive, evaluating, anticipating and choosing your decision carefully are all necessary if you are to trust your decisions and their appropriateness to your life and circumstances.

Evaluating your decisions for appropriateness is covered in more detail later in this chapter in "Steps to Proactive Decisions."

Aspect 4: Support

Good decisions involve making sure support exists for carrying them out. A good decision brings you into increasing contact with people who can help you widen your horizons and who can provide friendship as well as professional support. This need for support is one of the reasons a good decision must be appropriate to your life, and often to the others in your life, but there is a balance between finding support and making your decisions according to what other people think you should do.

If your family and friends are helpful, caring and respect your life decisions, they can constitute an excellent support system, but this is not always possible. If you are not surrounded by a good support team, it's necessary to build one because it will get you through times of self-doubt and difficulty, as well as motivate you and help you celebrate the good times.

Contacts with people and new ideas are important to your personal growth. When you learn to make decisions that maximize your opportunities for warm, stimulating relationships and new learning, you open up to everything good that will come to you from other people. So be wary of a decision that will lead to isolation. Joining a professional organization or a community-involved church increases your opportunities for personal growth and empowerment in decision making within the organization and provides a ready-made group of influential people who can help you meet your goals.

*To get her career as a counselor in private practice started, **Robin** needs to join professional organizations and get to know and talk to other counselors who have already been successful. Her church, alumni association and local activist groups working for human rights will be good* *sources for meeting successful counselors in the community. Because a private practice will require her to work in relative isolation, her decisions need to focus on balancing that with connections to the outer world through professional and social organizations. Through the counseling professionals she will meet in the organizations, she can get lots of the practical information about the business end of counseling that she feels she lacks.*

Megan*'s law office presents opportunities to talk with others at lunch and during and after work. Through the "employee grapevine" she can gather information to decide whether or not being a working mom is a good decision for her. If she decides to pursue her career full-time and forgo children for now, she can join employee organizations and enroll in job-related classes and workshops where she can get to know other successful women lawyers. An organization such as the Association of Women Trial Attorneys could provide priceless contacts with more experienced women who would be willing and able to mentor and help her in her career.*

*How much support is available on the job will be a factor for **Sharon** to consider if she receives a job offer in another state. Positive support at work, and an opportunity to socialize with coworkers, could help replace the social network of family and friends she would leave behind.*

If, like **Rita,** family is your main focus, you can join parenting groups, the PTA, a co-op nursery school or daycare center, and get connected with other parents. Rita got a great deal of help and good advice from meeting a group of working moms. Especially if you're a single mom, you'll find contact with other mothers reassuring and a great resource.

We'll see how all these women found, used and created support (and how you can, too) in chapter 8, "It Takes a Village."

Aspect 5: Self-Respect

A good decision will enhance your self-respect. Using your self-awareness, researching all the possibilities, making sure you have support to carry out your decision and making decisions appropriate to your life all contribute to making successful decisions. Sometimes, however, a decision that seems right on all those levels doesn't feel right for you. To make a decision that you can truly live with, you must be comfortable with the ethics and values it entails.

Kim faced this problem. While giving in to pressure from her family let her feel like an obedient daughter, devoting seven years of extremely demanding postgraduate work to a career she wasn't sure she wanted would have been very detrimental to her self-respect, not to mention that such demanding work, if she was really not motivated for her own reasons, would have been more than she could manage; and it probably would have led to failure.

Kisha, on the other hand, by turning her life around and getting herself educated and off welfare, has greatly increased her own level of self-respect; she has even given her children a more solid basis for their own self-images.

Life is an endless opportunity to make decisions. How you make them, to a large degree, determines how well your life will go, how much you will accomplish and how satisfied you will be with what happens. While none of us has complete control over what happens in life, how we react to what happens can make all the difference.

Reactive Versus Proactive

When observing women who feel they did not make good decisions in life, who are dissatisfied and unhappy, we often discover that they handled their lives in a reactive rather than a proactive way. Handling life reactively means waiting until something happens and then responding to it, often in an intuitive or emotional fashion, rather than thinking through your response beforehand.

Reacting

We all need to be able to react when something unforeseen happens, and often there is no time to do more than respond emotionally or intuitively. Consider the following examples:

- Your two-year-old child suddenly runs into the street. You immediately run after him, grab him and drag him back onto the sidewalk before you know what you are doing.

- Without thinking, you swerve the wheel of the car you are driving to miss an object in the road.

- Your best friend bursts into tears, and you put your arms around her and say, "There, there," before you even know what's wrong.

These are all appropriate reactive responses, and we use this wonderful ability to act without thinking or understanding many times a day. Most of the time it works. However, if you allow your immediate reactions to rule your life, you can find yourself in trouble. For example:

- You become repeatedly and disastrously involved with people who are destructive (that is, loving a charming but hopeless alcoholic, being taken in by a smooth sales rep, saying "yes" to an irresponsible sibling who wants to borrow your car).

- You spend money you can't afford (shopping when you're upset, loaning money to untrustworthy friends, renting a house that's too expensive because you love it).

- You behave in obsessive or addictive ways (overeating, getting drunk, working too many hours for little pay, overscheduling yourself).

Being Proactive

While your emotions are a good counterbalance for your intellectual analysis of a given situation; because how you feel about the person, situation or event may make you aware of subtle subconscious clues you're picking up; using emotional reaction as a substitute for rational decision making is usually a mistake. Important decisions must be made from the neck up as well as from the neck down. That is, each decision you make that will have a significant impact on your life should be considered intellectually as well as emotionally.

STEPS TO PROACTIVE DECISIONS

Proactive decisions are choices you make because you: (1) anticipate the need to choose, (2) evaluate the situation and your options, (3) choose a reasonable course of action based on your evaluation and (4) act on your choice.

This advice is not new. There are many aphorisms and proverbs that express the folk wisdom of proactive decisions: "A stitch in time saves nine." "Look before you leap." "Before running mouth, be sure brain is engaged." These expressions exist in our culture (as well as other cultures) because they are lessons that many people have found to be true. Whether from the Bible, Shakespeare, Benjamin Franklin, or a popular song, movie or play, the phrase catches on and is used repeatedly because it rings true.

Yet many women (and men, for that matter) fail to pay attention and think clearly enough to be proactive and decisive. You must be alert and aware to take action. The good news is it is not necessary to be proactive constantly; only when significant decisions need to be made. The 10 Smartest Decisions are examples of how being proactive now will save you a lot of work and hassle later.

Our first actions in a new situation set a pattern we are likely to follow for a long time. For example, when building a house or a fence, it's the first layer of bricks that must be laid with extreme care, including lots of measuring, leveling, etc., because all the other bricks laid will be affected by that first row.

Life decisions have that same effect. Once the basic decisions are made, you can often relax and follow through without thinking every other aspect through as carefully. The initial decisions act as a blueprint for your future actions, giving you a plan to follow. Unfortunately, this same phenomenon works in a negative sense, also. If your initial decisions are not well thought out, everything you do later follows the original flawed pattern and makes things worse.

Being proactive, then, is the first step to making good decisions. Once you decide to learn how to anticipate, evaluate, choose, and act wisely and effectively, essentially you are on the path to making the kinds of decisions that are right for you at each phase of your life.

Anticipate the Need to Choose

If you grew up in an authoritarian home, like Kim, or in a family that struggled through life but never learned how to take charge, like Kisha, or one where the "place" of women was to be loving, caretaking and responsive, you may have learned to focus on one or more people, taking your cues about what decisions to make from them. This trains you to be responsive and "outer directed" that is, to look for what to do from what is happening around you, rather than to generate your behavior from your own ideas. Women are often socialized in this fashion, which is the reason we are thought of as being sensitive, caring and understanding about others. (Of course, not all women are the same, and plenty of men are socialized in this way, too.)

If this is true for you, you may not be used to operating by thinking in advance about what might happen and getting prepared for it. Responsiveness is a very valuable skill to have, but it only works *after* there is something to respond to. Anticipation thinks ahead and plans for the unexpected as well as expected events and circumstances. Responsiveness is more a feeling, an intuitive and emotional response to a situation. Anticipation is more mental: thinking through the possibilities.

The problem side of anticipation is worry. If you anticipate what might happen, without figuring out what you can do about it, you'll just go around and around, getting more and more anxious: "What if my car breaks down?" "What if I don't get the job?" and so on. The way to avoid this is to treat the questions as genuine and to answer them: "If my car breaks down, I'll borrow some money and get it repaired." "If I don't get this job, I'll keep searching until I find one." Negative worrying can be turned into positive anticipation when it leads you to consider alternative possibilities and to plan for future events. If your anxiety level is so high that this "quick fix" doesn't work, or if you worry a lot, have anxiety attacks, or dread making decisions and being in charge, use the following checklist to help you turn your free-flowing anxiety into focused anticipation.

The Worrier's Guidelines

This exercise is especially effective when you can't sleep or when you experience anxiety attacks. If you worry a lot or obsess about future events and problems when you should be concentrating on other things, follow these simple steps:

1. **Write it down.** If you're feeling anxious or worried, or you can't stop thinking about some event that hasn't happened yet, take a few moments to write down whatever is worrying you. If you can't write it down, think it through carefully until you can clearly say what you're worrying about. Clarifying your worries will stop the free-floating sensation of anxiety with no basis.

2. **Evaluate.** Think about the first item on your list. Ask yourself, "Is there anything I can do about it now?" If you're at home and worrying about the office, or if the problem won't occur until next week or next year, you may not be able to do anything about it right now. Or, you may be worrying about something you could do something about, such as calling someone, or finding out how much something costs, or making a doctor's appointment to check out a worrisome symptom.

3. **Do something.** If there is something you can do, do it. Some- times, worry is a way to procrastinate. Often, worry is a way to keep a

mental list going, as in: "I'm worried that I'll forget to bring the slides for the presentation tomorrow."

- o *If you're worried about how your presentation will go at work tomorrow, go over your notes and lay out your clothes for the morning.*

- o *If you're worried about a health problem, look up the illness or*

- o *If you're at work and worrying about cooking dinner when you get home, write out a menu or a list of ingredients.*

- o *If you're worried that you may be fired, update your resume and call some employment agencies. You don't have to take another job, but if there's a real problem you'll be prepared.*

Here's an example: If you're worried that the roof may leak the next time it rains, start making a list about what you can do about it. Your inner dialogue may sound like this:

"The news said it was going to rain next week. I'm worried that the roof might leak."

"Call a roofing company and have them look at it."

"I'm worried that a roofing company will charge me more than it should because I don't know how much it should cost."

"Call my brother (or my neighbor, or my friend), who had his roof done, and ask him what it cost, and also if he liked the contractor he used."
"Okay."
When you reach this "okay," it's time to make the call, or if it's too late at night, to make a note to call the next day.

4.   **Distract yourself.** *When you've done what you can, or made your lists or notes, then distract yourself: Get busy doing something else, read, or take a walk or a bath.*

Repeat the above steps every time you catch yourself worrying.

If your personal history is full of unexpected catastrophes, unplanned hassles, and lots of anxiety and worry, you will benefit greatly from learning effective anticipation. To learn how to anticipate effectively, use the following checklist.

The Anticipation Exercise

Daily Anticipation: *Either in the evening or the morning, take fifteen to twenty minutes to sit down with your calendar and think about the day to come. Consider your to-do list, your appointments (whatever kind of appointments you have: with a business associate, a customer, your dentist, taking your child to soccer or ballet, or lunching with a friend) and whatever you personally would like to accomplish (for example, gardening, cooking dinner, writing your novel, working out, meditating or praying, creating art* or music, or visiting a friend). If your list is more than you can possibly accomplish in one day, sort through it now, instead of waiting until the end of the day to find you didn't accomplish the most important things. Prioritize what you have to do; and whatever you're not going to get to today, put on your to-do list for tomorrow or next week.

Look at your calendar and schedule as realistically as you can. For example, if you are taking your daughter to ballet class, consider that it might be important to allow enough time for the two of you to talk about some things that are bothering you or her. If the client you have to see is long-winded or habitually late, take that into consideration and find a way to cut it short, or use the wait time. If you are extra tired, consider not packing your day as full as usual.

On the other hand, if your calendar is not full enough, if you have a tendency to go to work and then come home with no idea of what you'll do for the evening, then give some thought to scheduling some of that unused time: volunteering to help somewhere, inviting a friend over, joining the church choir or taking a class, for example.

The point is to take charge of your day, and make sure that, within the limits of your situation, you do the things that are most important to you. The few minutes you take at the beginning of your day to organize it can save you hours later.

Kisha had a task calendar, but none at home: she would come home to chaos and confusion, and once the children were finally in bed she sat numbly in front of the TV. When she got herself a calendar to track her *personal time, she suddenly found it possible to plan ahead, help her children get organized, see friends and even get the laundry done every week. Having a personal schedule that she uses as effectively as the one at work means she can plan for household chores and help her children with homework and activities—and still make sure she gets some relaxation and recreation for herself. Anticipating the day's home chores, as she does the ones at work, means that she uses her time more effectively, gets the most important things done, and actually has extra time for taking classes and planning for the future. "I took a workshop given at work on organizing your day with a calendar planner— I knew how effective it was, but it took me awhile to catch on that it would be just as helpful at home," laughs Kisha. "I can't believe I waited so long to do it. It's a simple thing, but what a difference!"*

If you focus on planning each day, you will make steady progress toward attaining your future goals.

To start anticipating and planning for the future, begin dreaming about it. All plans begin as dreams, and the best plan for you will come from your own dreams, not those of your parents, spouse, boss or children. The overall plan may include any or all of the other people in your life, but you won't wholeheartedly follow through on your dream if you let others dictate it.

The Ten-Year Dream

To get in touch with your dream, record yourself reading the following guided fantasy very slowly and quietly, pausing to allow time to visualize, and play it to follow the prompts. Or, ask a friend to read it aloud to you.

Relax, breathe slowly and comfortably, get comfortable in your chair, and imagine that you're dreaming about your ideal life ten years from now. This is your life in ten years, if everything could happen just exactly the way you want it.

Now, with your eyes closed, and still in a relaxed state, let yourself wake up gently from the dream. It's morning on a day ten years in the future, and you're living a life that makes you completely happy. How do you wake up? To an alarm clock, to the sunlight, to what sounds or smells? What are your surroundings? Are you indoors? If so, what kind of bed and room are you in? Allow the colors, sounds and smells to register on your senses as you become more and more aware of your surroundings.

Now imagine gently getting up and getting ready to begin your day. What are you wearing? How are you getting ready? When you are ready to begin your day, move on to the next scene.

Where do you go next? Let each scene unfold, noticing the sights, sounds, smells and textures. Let yourself discover who is there with you and what you do at each hour of the day. Go as far as you want to from the place where you woke up, and notice what surrounds you. See yourself in your daily activities, alone or with other people, enjoying what you are doing. Take as much time

as you need to complete the day and to find out as
much about your life as you can.

When you finish the fantasy, write down a summary
of your experience. You can do this guided fantasy as
often as you want to discover more and more about your
ideal life. Talk about the characteristics of your ideal life
with the people closest to you. Allow yourself some time
to think about it, without arguing with it. Even if it seems
impossible to you today, let it be a dream for a while.

As you get more comfortable with your ideal,
consider how you could bring it, or parts of it, into
reality.

Allow yourself to anticipate your future as you expect
it to happen. If you have kids, imagine them growing up
and leaving home. What would you do then? Imagine
your next birthday. What would you like to be doing by
then? Imagine taking a class in something you'd like to
do: French, yoga, great books, creative writing, drawing
and painting, playing the stock market, or car mechanics.
Imagine completing the things you are working on now:
getting a raise, or completing your degree, or buying a
house, or paying off your mortgage, or starting your own
business. Imagining gives you a chance to anticipate
what you would do next, before you actually must make a
decision.

Evaluate the Situation

Positive anticipation will clarify what your options
are because you will consider in advance what needs to
be done, what you want to do, and what you have time to
do. The most desirable action is to blend the realities of

what you must do with your fantasy of what you want to do.

During your evaluation, you will answer a series of "what if" questions. The answers you come up with can vary from the fanciful to the practical—the ideal to the real. What's important is that you let yourself brainstorm a variety of possible scenarios and outcomes. I call this "playing chess" because the great chess masters continuously watch the board and project the possible effects of each move they could make. They may project many possible moves ahead of where they are to see which move is the best bet. Searching for as many possible options as you can find, gives you a better chance of coming up with your best answer.

Once your options are clear, you need to evaluate them to know which is the most effective. For example, you may want to live in a $500,000 house on a $30,000 per year income. There are several possible ways to resolve the disparity, from finding a way to change your income to choosing a cheaper house. What usually works best, however, is to examine all the options you imagined and decide what is important for you. You may want that house for status, because it's lovely to look at, because it's big enough for all your projects and friends, or because it overlooks the ocean. If you only require some of the components of the house: the ocean view, a front porch with columns, or more room than you have now, you may be able to get them in your price range. If you want the prestige, maybe you can get some of that by being active in your community. If it has to be *that* house, in *that* area, maybe you can start your own business, or become a real estate agent, and find a way to afford it.

The best way to evaluate the options is to check them against a list of requirements: Is it quiet enough, light and airy enough, close enough to work, within my price range, etc.?

The following list contains some suggested criteria for evaluating options:

- Is it practical?

- If it doesn't seem practical, is there a way you could make it practical, or are there some parts that are practical?

- What are the benefits?

- What are the drawbacks?

- Do you know the steps you have to follow to bring it about?

- How do the rewards (if it is successful) compare with the penalties (if it goes wrong)?

- Do you presently feel good about it?

- Does it make sense? Can you explain what you're doing clearly to someone else or on paper?

- Would you advise a friend to do it?

Making your own list of criteria, based on questions like these, will help you proactively evaluate your options.

Choose a Reasonable Course of Action

Surprisingly enough, once you have anticipated the event and evaluated the options, actually making the choice becomes simple. Because you have sufficient information, and you've evaluated the realistic aspects of your options, one or two best choices will stand out. Only if you have a rigid, dependent definition of the "right" way to do things, and are not open to considering new and different solutions, will your choice seem limited or blocked. For example, if it's cheaper, faster and less stressful to take the rapid transit system to work, but you insist that, for prestige, you have to drive in your Mercedes, your prejudice will prevent you from making the soundest, most effective choice.

If you have done the evaluation process thoroughly, a choice will usually become clear. If not, then you may need to do more research, ask some questions or talk to someone you trust who is experienced in similar matters.

Act On Your Choice

A choice is not really made until you act upon it. That is, if you have clearly decided what you think is the best thing for you to do under the circumstances, and you do not follow through, you have made a passive choice. Indecision, procrastination and denial are ineffectual ways to avoid the responsibility of making decisions. To act on your decision is to believe in it, to back yourself up. No one ever knows in advance if her decisions are right but, by proactively and thoughtfully making your own decisions, you raise the odds in your favor. Also, when you act on your decision, the action itself tests the decision, so that by paying attention to the results you can make new decisions as necessary.

If you find yourself unable to act on a decision, use that as a source of new information. Perhaps your decision did not take into account some aspect of your life or personality and needs to be reevaluated. Or perhaps you are trying to act on too much at once and need to break it down into smaller steps. As you go through The 10 Smartest Decisions in the following chapters, you will see how each can be acted upon effectively.

2
Don't Let Your Past Hold You Back: Decide to Resolve Old Issues

***

It would be very easy just to blame our parents and be victims for the rest of our lives. But that wouldn't be very much fun, and it certainly wouldn't get us out of our stuck position.

—Louise Hay

***

Making good decisions means being in charge of your own life. As long as unresolved issues from childhood, past relationships, difficult or unsuccessful career experiences, and other unfinished business are creating emotional upheaval in your life or your relationships, you will not be truly in charge. While it's very true that such experiences can be upsetting and emotionally very painful, allowing them to remain unresolved is to continue to decide *not* to be in charge of who you are or what your life is about.

HEALING A TROUBLED CHILDHOOD

There is no way to move your life along if you remain stuck in the past. However, "There is a way . . . to heal," writes psychologist Dr. Charles Whitfield in his celebrated book *Healing the Child Within*, ". . . and to break free of the bondage and suffering of our co-dependent or false self." If you were unlucky enough to have a difficult, unhappy or violent childhood, you need to do some work to overcome it, but that work is essential to the quality of the rest of your life.

The most beneficial thing you can do for yourself, and for those you love, is to face your past problems head on and do the work necessary to let go of the past hurts and get on with today. Do not get caught in the trap of thinking that there's nothing you can do to make things better. If your childhood was problematic, and your parents were too young, dysfunctional, addicted or violent, and you have not done the required work to resolve those problems, you are probably still treating yourself as badly as your parents treated you.

"Perhaps you were treated [badly] as a child, and that is sad," counselor and healer Louise Hay maintains in *You Can Heal Your Life*. "However, that was a long time ago, and if you are now choosing to treat yourself in the same way, then it is sadder still."

__Kisha__ became pregnant at sixteen and again at eighteen, partly because she was out of control on drugs and alcohol and partly because she hoped a baby would be someone to love her as her family had not. The social worker who supervised her welfare case got her into nearby Alcoholics Anonymous and Narcotics Anonymous programs and helped Kisha realize that she could have a better life for herself and her children. Her fear of losing her children if she remained addicted helped her stay focused on her recovery. Once she became clean and sober, she realized that she needed more help to work through her emotional problems, and she eventually was accepted into a treatment program that provided individual and group therapy.

Although some members of Kisha's family had accepted the same history she was replaying, others gave her the encouragement and emotional support she needed to change and grow, and she also found support within her church, which helped her survive the difficult years of recovery while raising two children on her own. Once she resolved the issues that were left over from her childhood, she was able to use the encouragement and support of her family and various groups to get training in computer science and a secure job. Kisha remembers, "It was really tough, and often scary, but the only way I could make myself and my kids secure was to let go of my past and the way my family had always done things."

Like Kisha, you can restructure your relationship to your family so that it becomes helpful rather than a hindrance.

OTHER LIFE TRAUMAS

Problems in your original family are not the only events that can be emotionally devastating to the point where they interfere in your life. Other life traumas include: automobile accidents or other injuries; serious illnesses; disability or death of a child, spouse, or parent; a personal disability or devastating illness; career or business failures; so-called acts of God (earthquakes, floods, tornadoes, etc.); a devastating divorce or relationship break-up; war or political exile; and care of aging parents or disabled family members.

All of these can leave lasting, devastating emotional scars that interfere with your natural intelligence and ability to make decisions. For a while after any of these events, it is natural to grieve, avoid life's smaller problems and seek refuge among the people you know. But if the emotional devastation lasts for an extended period of time, or is very strong, then counseling or a support group may be appropriate. Investing time and money now may make the difference in how well your life works in the future.

While teaching you how to heal your childhood wounds and the traumatic events of your life until now is beyond the scope of this book (See *It Ends with You: Grow Up and Out of Dysfunction* http://tinyurl.com/z6xafbv) I can and will suggest ways you might heal whatever traumatic experiences are in your way, and I will also tell you how to evaluate them to see if they are hampering your decision making.

THE POWER OF SELF-RESPECT

In the previous chapter, we learned that self-awareness is the first principle of good decision making. Fundamental to self-awareness is self-respect, because if you don't believe you are worthy of your own respect, you are not going to care enough about yourself to become objectively self-aware. If you lack self-respect, then the only self-awareness you may have is an on-going negative commentary on who you are and what you are doing.

Rita met her husband in high school, got married soon after and immediately became a mom. Because of this, she doubted that she had a personality and life of her own. Her whole life seemed to be about other people's needs. She constantly told herself that what she was doing was "all she could handle," and she felt bad when she heard that her high school friends were graduating from college, getting degrees and beginning careers. "I believed I was too stupid to do that," recalls Rita. "I didn't give myself credit for all the jobs I did at home, from keeping the budget and paying bills to all the psychological, emotional and practical skills involved in being a successful wife and mother."

She got a job for financial reasons but constantly worried that she wasn't good enough as a mother.

Past traumas can seriously undermine your self-respect, replacing it with feelings of low self-worth, shame, guilt or hopelessness. Such unhealed emotional wounds can also lead to behaviors that undermine your self-control, such as alcoholism, eating disorders, problems controlling your time and/or money, and dysfunctional relationships with people in both your private and business life.

Rita eventually began to feel worse and worse, sleeping poorly, having trouble getting up in the morning, and developing headaches and other mysterious physical symptoms. Her doctor did tests and told her there was nothing physically wrong, but he thought it might be stress-related. After resisting for a couple of years, Rita finally took his advice and found a therapist. "She helped me see that I'm bright and competent enough to make a success of anything I want to do," Rita explains. "She showed me that my fears came from my parents, who loved me but treated me (and each other) in a critical, belittling style that made me think I wasn't good enough."

Marriage and motherhood were a wonderful challenge at first, but they eventually became a place to hide. Rita resolved her old family issues and was ready to try some new things. She began to dream some dreams and to take the first steps to make them come true.

Signs that unresolved issues might be a problem for you include the following:

Depression: If you function okay most of the time, but your mood is somber, you cannot get to sleep at night, you have trouble waking up and getting going in the morning, you feel mentally "fuzzy" a lot of the time, or you are very discouraged and hopeless, you could be suffering from a light to moderate case of clinical depression. Getting therapy to resolve old issues could make a huge difference in your life. Don't let any doctor prescribe any mood-altering drugs without adjunctive therapy, because, unsupported, drugs may eventually make the problem worse. Instead, find a qualified Licensed Clinical Social Worker, Licensed Counselor or Therapist, or Licensed Clinical Psychologist and begin therapy, which may include medication. Research shows that the combination of medication and therapy is best for depression and/or anxiety.

Anxiety: If you have panic attacks during which your heart flutters, your breathing becomes rapid and you feel overwhelmed with fear, or if you are worried and anxious most of the time, these conditions also can be caused by unresolved feelings from the past. Anxiety is quite easy to fix with the help of a competent counselor.

Addictive, Obsessive or Compulsive Behavior: If your life feels out of control and you are using alcohol or drugs (prescription or not) to excess; misusing food by binging and purging or starving yourself; compulsively spending and in debt; or trapped in a destructive relationship, you won't be able to make the decisions you need to make unless you take care of the problem first. Find a self-help group such as Alcoholics Anonymous www.aa.org, Overeaters Anonymous www.OA.org, or Adult Children of Alcoholics www.ACA.org, and perhaps a treatment and detox program to help free yourself of these problems.

Unresolved Grief: If you have had losses in your life that you have not sufficiently grieved, the unexpressed grief can stop you from moving on. If you try to avoid feeling the emotions and the loss, the grief will remain unresolved. If you have lost a loved one, such as a spouse, child, parent, close relative or dear friend (or even a beloved pet), or your home or an important job, or have had some disability or disease that drastically changed your life, the appropriate response is to grieve. If you don't know how or are unable to feel those feelings, or you're not supported in doing so by the people around you, therapy or a grief group can be immensely helpful in finishing up, letting go and moving on with your life.

Rage: If you are frequently angry and frustrated, lack patience and have emotional outbursts, you may be dealing with anger left over from the past. Again, individual or group therapy can help you resolve your rage and regain control of your life.

Procrastination or Feeling Blocked: If you are unable to follow through on the things you decide to do or unable to make decisions, you may be blocked by an unresolved issue from the past. Rather than push yourself to do what you want to do, take the time to create a journal or talk to a friend or a counselor about your feelings. Depression, anxiety, compulsions, grief and/or rage can all act as "blockers" that tie up so much of your energy you are too drained to act. If you write or talk about your feelings rather than the plans or activities you are unable to accomplish, you will uncover a feeling that can be resolved.

Burnout: Women often experience burnout after several years of parenting, working in a helping career (such as teaching, nursing, and legal and medical fields) or just working a difficult job. Burnout is not unusual in a demanding career, but taking good care of yourself often can prevent it. Again, therapy can be well worth the time and money invested.

Sleep Problems: Disturbing dreams, anxiety, depression and other symptoms of unresolved issues can make it difficult to sleep soundly and for enough hours to maintain optimum health. Like burnout, sleep problems can be a sign of early issues that need attention. Rather than asking your doctor for sleeping pills, which can be very addictive and have side effects, some people have found therapy, hypnosis and biofeedback effective remedies for curing sleep problems.

Mysterious Health Problems: If you have back or other chronic pain, digestive problems, frequent headaches or other health problems for which your doctor is unable to find a cause, the symptoms may be the result of tension caused by unresolved trauma. Again, try therapy, hypnosis or biofeedback to uncover the root of the tension, which you then can resolve.

Ongoing Family Problems: If your parents or your siblings are taking an unreasonable amount of your time and energy, either because they upset you often, or they ask a lot of you that they could be doing themselves, or they are constantly creating problems in your life, you are probably still relating to them as you did in childhood and you need to "grow up" in relationship to your childhood family. If, on the other hand, it's your husband and children who are giving you problems and not being responsible, you are probably relating to them in a way that is patterned on your early family. Either way, family or individual therapy to sort out your intimate relationships will teach you how to focus on what's important in your life and how to keep your family, your personal life and your professional life in balance. On the other hand, if your parents require a lot of care because they're elderly or infirm, or someone else needs extra care because of a serious illness or disability, that is a real-life condition, not a holdover from childhood, and it must be managed. How to manage it will be discussed later in this chapter.

Struggles with Coworkers or Other Work Relationships: We often encounter difficult people at work, but if you seem to have more difficulty with your coworkers than others do, or if you have had problems on several jobs, then old issues are spilling over into your work life, and therapy is again the answer.

By searching online, you will find referral sources for the therapies and resources suggested above. If any of the symptoms described are problems for you, the best thing you can do for yourself is to resolve them now, the sooner the better, even if it seems to postpone your other plans for a while.

HEALTHY FAMILY RELATIONSHIPS

What is the difference between healing old wounds and becoming stuck in them? The preceding list is a dramatic argument for the importance of healing old wounds. If any such symptoms apply to you, then you are stuck emotionally to some degree: reliving the trauma over and over. This indicates there is work to be done about your original family and your childhood or about trauma that occurred after childhood. When you are focusing on these old incidents in order to express and resolve the emotions, you are healing the wounds. If your family wounds are deep or painful, you will probably need help, as suggested above.

Even if such symptoms don't apply to you, many of us have other difficulties moving past our childhood relationships with family to new, adult and equal-status connections. Parents frequently have trouble letting go of children and seeing them as independent adults. Whether you're twenty, thirty or older, you may still be "Little Mary" or "Big Sis" to your parents and siblings. It's really up to you to change your relationship with your family until it's healthy for you as an adult.

But what is a healthy family? Most of us are familiar with the term "dysfunctional family" and know it means a family with problems, but did you know that the opposite of a dysfunctional family is a functional family? The terms arose from the fact that every family has functions it needs to perform.

Dysfunctional families do not emotionally support the participants, foster communication among them, appropriately challenge them, or (especially in the case of families of origin) prepare or fortify them for life in the larger world. In short, they are families or relationships that do not effectively enhance the lives of the people involved and don't function as they should. People in these relationships don't take responsibility for making their own lives or relationships work, and they may take too much responsibility for others.

The degree of dysfunction in a relationship or family can vary. Most of us get a little dependent, and therefore dysfunctional, from time to time: especially when we're tired, stressed or otherwise overloaded. The difference between this normal, occasional human frailty and true clinical dysfunction is our ability to recognize, confront and correct dysfunction when it happens in our relationships.

> **Kim** *was born into an immigrant family with strong beliefs about maintaining family ties and traditions. Because of this, Kim believed that she must do everything just the way her parents wanted. Her family loves her very much and wants the best for her. They made a lot of sacrifices so that their daughter could be a doctor. Kim, however, was having second thoughts as she knows how tough medical school will be. She didn't know if she wanted to do this for herself, for her family or at all. But she was afraid to tell them this because she didn't want to disappoint them. One day, her grandmother said, "Kim, you don't look happy. What is wrong?" Because her grandmother is wise, loving and forgiving, Kim was able to talk*

about her fears. True to form, Grandmother said, "I know your parents want great things for you, and so do I. But most of all, we all want you to be happy. So you must figure out what you want to do." With that support, Kim was able to talk to her family about whether a medical career will really work for her.

The question to keep in mind is this: What is not working, and how can I make it work? Most people, when faced with a relationship problem or disagreement, reflexively look for a villain; that is, they want to know who's at fault. Responding to a problem by looking for someone to blame (even if it's yourself) is a dysfunctional response. The functional question is not, "Whose fault is it?" but, "What can I do to solve the problem?"

When you try it, you'll see that refusing to focus on blaming anyone (yourself, a family member or your partner), and insisting instead on solving the problem, will make a huge difference in all your relationships. Families who sit together in a family meeting where everyone, including small children, gets to discuss a problem from their point of view, and everyone works together to solve the problem, rapidly become more functional. Direct communication is more functional than indirect communication. You can make the communication in your family of origin more direct by not being willing to listen to complaints or gossip about other family members ("I think this is John's personal life you're telling me about, and I'd rather not discuss it.") and by not carrying messages from one family member to another ("If you want mother to know you're hurt, please tell her yourself.").

Family members or couples who can sit together and discuss problems calmly, without blaming, criticizing or accusing, find that looking for a mutual solution to their problems increases their commitment and intimacy and bonds them together. Nothing binds you in relationship more powerfully than the awareness that by working together you can solve whatever problems arise.

NO FAMILY IS PERFECT

No relationship will be perfect, and how to successfully interact cannot be worked out in advance. What you can do is learn basic communication techniques, build your self-esteem, and develop patterns for healthy, equal, and balanced loving on your own, which will help you make your relationship with your family of origin or your own partner and children much more successful. If they affect you negatively and you cannot change what goes on, you may find it necessary to limit your involvement with certain family members or in certain family interactions. This can be done subtly and with kindness, if you plan it carefully. You can still be pleasant with the uncle who is alcoholic and becomes abusive when he's drunk; you simply avoid his presence when he begins to drink, even at functions where this usually happens (like a family wedding). It's a lot healthier (and easier) to focus on those family members who are pleasant and fun to be around and to limit your conversations with troubled family members to brief, polite exchanges about the weather or other superficial topics.

THE TIME OUT

No matter how acceptable your family may think they are, you can decide that certain behaviors are not acceptable to you, such as the following:

- drunkenness or a drugged state

- abusive or obnoxious language

- rage and yelling

- physical violence toward people or objects

- inappropriate sexual innuendos and advances

- mean and belittling comments, either to you or behind your back

- socially unacceptable actions, such as displays of bigotry or racism or

- embarrassing behavior of any kind (especially if repeated).

If anyone persists in behaving in these ways in your presence, using the time-out technique is a powerful and subtle way of fixing the problem. Modern parents know that one of the best ways to discipline a small child is to give him or her a *time out*: Send the child to a corner, or a room, all alone, until he or she has thought about the problem, then discuss the issue and resolve it. What you may not realize is that time outs work great, too, on any adult who is acting childish or misbehaving. All you need to do is become distant but polite around anyone—in your family, at work, at school, or among your friends—who is not treating you well. There is no need to tell the person what you are doing: He or she will get the message from your behavior—which is much more effective. If you've never tried this, you'll be amazed at how effective becoming polite and pleasant but distant can be. Most of the time, the other person's behavior will immediately become more subdued around you and, often, much more caring. Eventually, that person may ask you what's wrong, or why you've changed. At that point (and only at that point) you have an opportunity to tell him or her what the problem behavior is and why you don't like it.

Your family can be a test case. If you can learn enough poise and finesse to extract yourself from dysfunctional or unpleasant encounters with family members without making matters worse, you will be better equipped to deal with anyone else in your life who gets out of line. Learning to put obnoxious people in time outs right at the beginning of unpleasant behavior can make it unnecessary to use tougher tactics at all.

BALANCING YOUR FEELINGS, NEEDS AND WANTS WITH OTHERS

With those members of your family who behave appropriately but who may want more from you than you can give, it is essential to learn to keep your needs and wants balanced with theirs. If you understand that, to be successful, your family relationships must be healthy and satisfying for everyone involved, you also understand that habitually putting others' feelings, needs and wants before your own is as harmful as compulsively putting your own wants, needs and feelings before anyone else's.

When people you care about ask you for help, support, comfort, care, errand running, etc., take a moment to make sure the request is reasonable. Elderly parents or grandparents or an ill sibling, spouse, or child may make demands on your time very appropriately (see the Aging Parents section later in this chapter.) However, most families have a member or two who seem incapable of doing things for themselves, or who always seem to ask for a lot more than they give. If such a person should, by all indications, actually be capable of handling the problems themselves, then it is highly detrimental to you to be giving time and resources you can't afford. The same is true for relatives whose lives are out of control because of some addiction, mental illness or other problem that needs treatment.

Devoting time and attention to people who really need to take care of themselves or to be in some kind of treatment can distract you from your life goals and make it impossible to make your own life work, which will harm you and everyone else you care about. Your family can learn to solve such issues and problems together through honest and open communication, and you can learn to achieve a balance. That is, you can work together to make sure all of you get your needs and wants met, and you can all care equally about your mutual satisfaction, health and happiness. If most of your family members understand this, you can work together to contain any of those who don't and to confront them in a loving way with their passivity, neediness or need for treatment.

Any other definition of love tends to degenerate into dysfunction and will become toxic to you and your family or partner. In a healthy family, finding out if solutions are mutually satisfactory is easy: You ask each other how it feels.

Changing your relationship with your family is much easier and more pleasant than you may believe. I invite you to consciously move your focus from who's at fault to what will fix the problem, to increase the mutuality and communication in your relationship, and to watch whatever dysfunctional interaction you have, whether it's mild or severe, be significantly reduced.

CREATING AN ADULT FAMILY RELATIONSHIP

To change your relationship with your family from that of a dependent child to a fully respected adult, you must first change the way you think of yourself in relationship to your family. In other words, to stop being treated as you were when you were a child, you must stop behaving the way you did as a child. If you treat others in your family as "fellow adults," you're more likely to get treated like one yourself. The ways your family members interact are just habits, and they can change. Following are some guidelines.

Guidelines for Growing Up Within Your Family

1. **Call your parents "Mother" and "Father" or "Mom" and "Dad," instead of childlike names such as Mommy, Daddy, Poppy, etc.** *It will make you think differently about your interaction.*

2. **Change your conversation to be more like the conversations you have with friends.** *Don't limit it strictly to family memories, or gossip about family members, or questions about your personal life. Before you speak with family members, take a minute to think of what "adult" topics you'd like to talk about. Current events, sports, work issues (just facts and events—avoid com plaining), political or local neighborhood issues are all adult topics.*

3. **If you have children of your own, share with your parents on a parent-to-parent basis.**

4. **Don't react if your parent does or says something annoying.** *Just ignore it and change the subject.*

5. **Don't ask your parents for advice—***try offering your own expertise instead—but offer it as you would to a friend. Don't push.*

6. **Pay attention to the balance of your interaction.** *Don't let your role slide into all giving or all receiving; try to keep the score even, as you probably do with your friends.*

7. **In general, treat your parents and siblings as if they were the family of someone you care about, and not your own**. *After all, if you were with a friend's family and someone did something odd, you'd ignore it and wouldn't let yourself be drawn into family squabbles: you'd be polite and pleasant, for your friend's sake.*

After following these guidelines for a few months, your interactions with your family will change so that you can relax and truly be your adult self. You'll find that families are more fun after you leave your childhood behavior patterns and left over emotions behind.

AGING PARENTS

If your parents are elderly and becoming infirm, or if others in your family require special care because of disability or illness, the situation is different. Family members who need help, whether they are acting appropriately or not, cannot be abandoned.

The major problem with such situations is that you have to figure out how to maintain a balance between the rest of your life and this often taxing situation. If you have a large family, sharing the responsibilities often lightens the burden of care, but if you are an only child, the problem will be more difficult to resolve.

It is beyond the scope of this book to go into all the details necessary to discuss proper care of the elderly or those who are seriously ill, but you must take charge of your own life and not let it be all about the past or your family members. The following guidelines will help you make the appropriate decisions to help those in need, while keeping your own life functional.

Guidelines for Helping Family Members in Need

1. **Get as much information as you can.** *Learn what the problem is, what kind of help is needed and what is involved in the care. Often local agencies, such as a senior citizens center or a nonprofit foundation for the particular disease or disability involved, will have lots of good information. The Internet is also an amazing source for finding help. Search for "Senior Care" or "Help for Elderly" and find resources in your area.*

2. **Make sure your entire family knows what the problem is and what kind of help is needed.** *Don't let reluctance to "bother" people or to tell the truth, or an old family relationship problem, get in the way of utilizing all the help that everyone in the family can give. If you have five people who can share the care and help, you'll obviously have an easier time than if you try to do it alone.*

3. **Work to find a way for each family member to contribute in the way that works best for him or her.** *As long as the burden feels fairly distributed in general, don't worry if one member contributes more time and another more money. It all qualifies as help, and if you try to make everyone do the same thing, you'll end up in a struggle.*

4. **Have regular discussions among the caregivers.** *Discuss how the arrangements are working, if everyone is doing his or her share, and how everyone feels about it. Clearing the air frequently will prevent resentments from piling up. Paid caregivers may be included in planning discussions.*

5. **Use community resources.** *Especially if you're alone, use as many community resources as you can find. People often feel negative about senior care residences or convalescent hospitals, but if placing your family member in a care facility is financially workable and it relieves the burden of actual care so that you can be more emotionally supportive, that may well be a good decision. If your family member is at home, make sure you check out home health or hospice care options with your doctor, your medical insurance and community agencies.*

6. **Find support for yourself.** *If you are doing this jointly with other family members, use your*

family meetings as times to air your frustrations and feelings and to support each other. If you are caring for a loved one by yourself, let your friends know you'll need a lot of emotional support and allow them to help.

7. **Take breaks whenever you can.** *This kind of care is very stressful. If you can manage to get away occasionally (one day a week, or when the visiting nurse comes in, or rotating weekends off if you have help), you'll be mo re able to handle the day-to-day pressure.*

MOVING ON

If you're over eighteen and in college, working or married, it's time to grow up and move on from your family and your childhood. While it's lovely to be close to your family if you have a good relationship with them, it is also time to build a life of your own, and the sooner you begin, the quicker you will become well-established. It's a big change when you first leave home to think of yourself as being in charge of your life. As Rita said, "I'm thirty-one years old, and I still feel as if someone else is running my life."

The key is to decide that you and only you are in charge of what you do from this day on. You can discuss your life issues with your parents, siblings, spouse and friends and make use of their experience and differing viewpoints; but in the end, you are the one who must make the decisions about what to do. Even if you manage to allow someone else to make the decisions for you, you will have to live with the consequences of those decisions. Following is a guided fantasy I use to help me make both big and small decisions.

The Wise Woman Exercise

In this guided fantasy, designed to help you achieve a helpful perspective on your own future, you create an advisor for your life decisions. Record the following, very slowly and quietly, and play it back, or ask a friend to read it aloud to you:

Relax, breathe slowly and comfortably, get comfortable in your chair, and picture a woman of seventy or more. This woman is just the kind of older woman you admire, the one you would like to be "when you grow up." She is financially secure, in good health, surrounded by people who care about her, good friends and family... She has lots of interests to keep her busy, and she stays active, which keeps her healthy, and happy... Introduce yourself to this woman ... As she gives you her name, you notice it's the same as yours... She is you, later in life... Make an agreement with this ideal older self that you will get advice from her about what decisions you need to make, as life goes on, to live to her healthy and happy state of being. Continue your conversation with her for as long as you wish and ask her what her secret is for living to such a lovely old age.

Check out your decisions regularly, by using your "wise woman." For example, how does this inner counselor react to your choice of a career? At her age, will you look back on it and think it was worth it? What about your choice of a spouse? Does your elder self approve? Does she think your choice will last? What is the difference between what you regard as important and what she regards as important?

Your inner "wise woman" is a very effective tool to help you look at your own life and your decisions from a different and valuable perspective. The decisions you make today affect the rest of your life, and you are ultimately the only person to whom you are accountable and for whom you are responsible. Every new decision is truly a new life's resolution. You'll also use your wise woman to help you sort out the third decision, your road map, in the next chapter.

3
Where Are You Going?
Decide to Set Realistic Goals and Priorities

*Luck is a matter of preparation
meeting opportunity.*

—Oprah Winfrey

In the previous chapters, we discussed the five basic aspects of decision making (self-awareness, research, appropriateness, support and self-respect); the four steps to proactive decisions (anticipate, evaluate, choose and act); and how to resolve old issues from the past and move on to being in charge of your own life. Armed with these principles and steps, you are ready to evaluate your own life from where you are now and to begin to shape it the way you want it. As Marsha Sinetar says in *Ordinary People as Monks and Mystics*, "To find in ourselves what makes life worth living is risky business, for it means that once we know it we must seek it. It also means that without it life will be valueless."

THE POWER OF LONG-RANGE GOALS

Let's pretend you are in a small, provincial town and you don't like it, but you don't know where you would like to be. As long as you don't know where you're going, you will either be stuck where you are or wandering aimlessly (meandering might be nice for a vacation, but it won't really tell you where you want to be). However, the following will happen if you use the principles of sound decisions:

- Through self-awareness, you'll realize you don't want to be where you are.

- Through research (which could include some wandering), you'll discover some other nice places to be.

- Through appropriateness, you'll compare places to find the right ones for you.

- Through support, you'll get the encouragement and cooperation you need to make the choice.

- Through self-respect, you'll determine it's the right decision for you.

You can systematically work out the details: such as whether you'd like to be in a bigger city, a warmer climate, etc.; until you have enough information to know where you want to go.

Once you have made a decision, you are instantly empowered to carry it out. For example, if you want to get from a small town in Iowa to San Francisco, California, many of your future decisions are already made. If you make the decisions that take you closer to San Francisco, you'll get there.

Simple as this sounds, life decisions are often the same. From a small decision, such as wanting a new outfit, to a giant decision, such as whether or not to have children, once you have chosen the major direction, a lot of decisions are essentially made for you. This makes life easier and your choices clearer. For example, if, in high school, you know you want to go to college and you want to get a teaching credential eventually, then the choices of your high school classes are mostly made according to the requirements of the colleges you would like to attend.

After I made the decision at age twenty-eight to leave my career as an accountant and go back to school to get a master's degree in psychology and a license as a psychotherapist, most of my subsequent choices were pre-determined for the next six years, and many of my choices today are facilitated by having made that decision.

Long-range goals are decisions that are going to affect your life for years to come. You don't need to know all the details to make a long-range decision: in fact, knowing all the details is usually not possible.

*When **Kisha** made her decision to get off welfare, do things differently than her mother and sisters had done, and make a more secure life for her* *children, it had an enormous effect on everything she has done since. She has made hundreds of smaller decisions since then, from what to buy for groceries, to daycare and schools for her children and herself, all of which were shaped by that first decision. "I had no way of knowing what would happen, or even if I would succeed—but I did know what I wanted." Kisha explains that each time she faced a choice, she evaluated it in light of her long-range plan. "I made many big and small sacrifices along the way and faced some tough choices, but my dream and my plan to make it come true sustained me and kept me motivated." Knowing she had a goal made it easier to stay focused on her future.*

SETTING YOUR OWN PRIORITIES

According to Webster's dictionary, a priority is "something which must be done or taken care of first," but who gets to decide which of the many things you might do is a priority? If you have decided to decide, as we discussed in chapter 1, you set your own priorities. While these may take others' wants and needs into account, the final authority in your life must be you. So, fundamental to establishing a "road map" for your plan is learning to set your own priorities.

If, whenever you need to, you can rapidly make a list of what is most important to you, you have learned to set priorities. Your list may vary according to whether you are focusing on the next hour, the whole day, the week, the year or many years. For example, if an appointment is canceled and you suddenly have a free hour, can you decide immediately how you'll use it, or does the hour go by before you have figured out what you want to do?

It helps to consider your priorities in descending order, that is, the overall priorities for your life in general, down to the more detailed priorities of the moment. Once you have decided what your central focus is, you narrow your choices, much like deciding to eat only vegetarian meals limits how many decisions you must make when you look at a restaurant menu.

YOUR MAIN PRIORITY

Knowing what you want your life to be about will limit your endless and overwhelming options in a similar way. What is most important to you? Do you want a career, a marriage, children or a loving relationship without children? Do you want your life to be about art, or achievement, or family or helping people? While some of us are very clear on that issue from a pretty early age, others feel confused about what they really want for most of their lives. Satisfaction comes only when you know what you want and you manage to achieve at least some of it.

In *Peace, Love and Healing*, Dr. Bernie Siegel writes, "Whatever your age, if you learn to listen, your inner voice will speak to you about your path . . . your 'job on earth.' . . . This wisdom that is directing you from within is your birthright . . . an inner message, an inner awareness, that says, 'This is your path, this is how you can be the best human being possible.' If you follow it, you will achieve your full growth and full potential as a human being before you let go of the Tree of Life."

GOALS AND MOTIVATION

If you don't know what is important to you, you can never get to the point of feeling that you've achieved your goals. Without goals, life becomes much like running a race with no finish line. Unless your goal is the running itself (which can be a very satisfying way of life) you never get to celebrate winning even the shortest race. If, on the other hand, you set goals for yourself, even small ones, you get to have many moments of satisfaction and celebration. It is from this celebration and recognition of having achieved a goal that most of us find the motivation to go on to the next goal. Thus, the "success equation" becomes celebration + appreciation = motivation. Following are three exercises you can do to help set your main priority.

Priority Exercise 1: The Questions

Answer these questions, and then use the answers to do the next exercise.

1. *What do you most like to do?*

2. *What makes you happy?*

3. *What gives you a feeling of satisfaction?*

4. *What productive activity would you do if you didn't need to be paid?*

5. *Do you prefer being around lots of people, a few people, one person or being alone?*

6. *When you are an old woman, what life accomplishments will you feel good about?*

7. *Rank, in the order of importance to you (most important being first) the following list:*

- *financial success*

- *career*

- *helping people*

- *immediate family*

- *extended family*

- *artistic expression*

- *self-expression*

- *physical activity*

- *spiritual or religious observance*

- *emotional expression*

- *communication*

- *intimacy*

- *sexual satisfaction*

- *having children*

- *love*

8. *Using the above list as a guide, make your own list of what is important to you.*

Priority Exercise 2: Your Job on Earth

Try this exercise if your main priority eludes you, you feel confused or overwhelmed by life, or if your life seems to lack meaning or an important reason for your existence.

Since each of us is unique, with different genetic mixes, different fingerprints, different gifts and personalities, let's suppose that there must be a reason—a plan—for our uniqueness. Included in the plan is a special place for each of us, and we have been designed, by a Super Intelligence, for a special task within the plan. What is your part in that plan? What were you designed to do? What's your "job on earth?"

Imagine: you are God and you created the human being that is you. What have you created that person for? The clues reside in your unique characteristics. If you assume that the secret to your life's purpose is hidden in your heart's desire, then by discovering your innermost wants, you can also find meaning, joy and purpose.

Are you a good listener? Maybe counseling people in some capacity is your intended "job." Are you a mathematical whiz? A musician? An artist? Can you make people laugh? Each of these talents can be used in unique ways to make the world a little better. For example, if you like to make people laugh and you enjoy elderly people, perhaps entertaining, volunteering, or working in a senior citizens' center is your special place. If you are a survivor of abuse or illness, perhaps your purpose lies in helping others survive.

The clues and hints are subtle, but they exist. Use your answers to the questions in Priority Exercise 1 to discover them.

The philosopher Joseph Campbell wrote in *The Power of Myth*, "If the person insists on a certain program, and doesn't listen to the demands of his own heart, he's going to risk a schizophrenic crackup. Such a person has put himself off center. He has aligned himself with a program for life, and it's not the one the body's interested in at all. The world is full of people who have stopped listening to themselves or have listened only to their neighbors to learn what they ought to do, how they ought to behave, and what the values are that they should be living for."

In my experience, as women find their sense of purpose regarding what they were "intended" to do or be, they feel as if they have joined the rhythm of a Super Intelligence and life begins to make more sense, doubt fades, and joy becomes a more frequent companion. Listen to your heart and to what is obvious about you: it works. Here's Dr. Campbell's advice about how to begin:

"You must have a room, or a certain hour or so a day, where you don't know what was in the newspapers that morning, you don't know who your friends are, you don't know what you owe anybody, you don't know what anybody owes to you. This is a place where you can simply

experience and bring forth what you are and what you might be. This is the place of creative incubation. At first, you may find that nothing happens there. But if you have a sacred place and use it, something eventually will happen... Where is your bliss station? You have to try to find it. Get a phonograph and put on the music that you really love, even if it's corny music that nobody else respects. Or get the book you like to read. In your sacred place you get the 'thou' feeling of life . . . for the whole world. I even have a superstition that has grown on me as a result . . . that if you do follow your bliss you put yourself on a kind of track that has been there all the while, waiting for you, and the life that you ought to be living is the one you are living. When you can see that, you begin to meet people who are in the field of your bliss, and they open the doors to you. I say, follow your bliss and don't be afraid, and doors will open where you didn't know they were going to be."

If you dare to get acquainted with your heart's desire, you can follow your bliss. By making a resolution to surrender, to slow down, you can find out what is inside straining to get out, longing to make contact with you. Make a "sacred space" for yourself and spend a little time in it, at first reading or listening to music, and little by little listening to your heart. If you do, you will discover what your main priority is.

Priority Exercise 3: Consulting Your Wise Woman

Consulting with your inner "wise woman," as we discussed in the previous chapter, is one way to sort out your overall life priorities. What goals, assuming you'll reach them, will give you satisfaction when you get to the age of your wise woman? At that stage of your life, what will seem important to you? What will not seem worth the effort? Having a long discussion with your elder advisor about what she thinks your life is all about can be very helpful in setting your priorities.

When **Megan** realized that her law career could cut her off from having children and spending time with them, she experienced a crisis. She loved her work and enjoyed the challenge of the law, but she also felt that corporate law was relatively meaningless, although it was very lucrative. Doing the above exercises led Megan to realize that both family and career are important to her, but beyond that she needed to feel as if she were making a difference in the world. She researched the various kinds of law she might practice and decided to work for a nonprofit agency to help battered and abused women and children. Her work environment in that concerned agency includes a daycare facility and more flexible hours, so Megan is getting serious with a suitable man who wants to have a family and they are planning for marriage and children. Her fiancé understands that Megan wants to continue work, and her employer understands that she plans to have a family. "Having both career and children may not be easy, but it is possible," believes Megan, "and I know I will feel more fulfilled as a woman and a mother by doing both."

INNER AND OUTER PRIORITIES

If you find the previous exercises difficult, or if they make you anxious, consider that you might be experiencing a conflict between inner and outer priorities.

As you probably discovered when doing these exercises, there are many different kinds of priorities, and often they conflict with each other. We have many kinds of needs: the basic survival needs such as food, shelter, and human connections, and the more complex, higher-level needs such as self-expression, emotional satisfaction, freedom from political and social oppression, pleasure, accomplishment, and positive reinforcement. Unless these needs are met, any of them can become a life priority.

These needs can be divided roughly into two categories: inner needs and outer needs. The concrete tangible needs for shelter and sustenance, financial security, other people, the trappings of success, recognition from others, etc., are outer needs, and those you feel most strongly about will become your outer priorities. The more intangible, invisible needs, such as emotional connection, self-esteem, fulfillment, personal freedom, happiness, and satisfaction, are your inner needs, and those you feel most strongly about will become your inner priorities.

Inner and outer priorities are often in conflict. For example, you may have a strong need for lots of personal freedom (an inner priority) and at the same time have a strong need for recognition in the community (an outer priority) which means you need to conform to community standards. That conflict can produce anxiety.

If you feel anxious over developing your road map, take some time to explore your thoughts and find out if you have a connection between inner and outer priorities.

The connection between what brings you satisfaction and what the outside world requires of you is complex, and a conflict between them is not easily solved. **Megan** feels an inner priority to be a mother and have a family and an outer priority to have a successful career. Because she was willing to become aware of her feelings and to consider every alternative she could, Megan found a very fine solution that satisfied both of her priorities. It also required her to sacrifice something: her salary is a lot less than as a corporate lawyer. However, since money is a lower priority for Megan, she has been able to make that sacrifice quite easily.

THE BALANCING ACT

Priorities are not set in concrete: They grow, diminish, move, and change with your life circumstances, your experience, and your maturity. No priority is always at the top of your list. As we discussed at the beginning of this chapter, there are priorities of the moment, of the hour, of the day, the week, the year and for your entire lifetime. For now, motherhood is a priority for Megan, but once she has her children and they begin school she will have more time and energy to focus on her career. "Being there for my children, once I have them, will be my top priority, and that will not change," explains Megan, "but as my children go to school, they will need me less and I will have more time for myself, and more flexibility. However, if one of my children is ill, or upset, as long as I am needed, being Mom will again be right at the top of the list."

As long as you have more than one priority (and everyone does), you must learn to do a balancing act. Career success may be important, and on the day you're dealing with a big client it may be more important than anything, including your family, or your own health (you make the presentation even though you're not feeling well). If you suddenly get a severe case of the flu, however, or your child does, then that takes precedence.

The most important thing about your balancing act is that you keep the end result in mind. Yes, it is very possible to have greater and lesser priorities, along with inner and outer priorities, and to keep them all active. What makes it possible to keep your lifetime priorities in focus is to recalibrate periodically to ensure that all the most important priorities are on track. Megan will need to constantly review and reassess to make sure her focus on mothering doesn't get lost in her work, and vice versa, and also that her own well-being doesn't get neglected in pursuit of her other priorities. This may sound difficult, but she can do it almost automatically if she develops a habit of making sure all the parts of her plan are getting the attention they need. She learned to use the following exercise to help her stay in balance.

Daily Balance Exercise

Once you get used to doing this exercise, you will be able to do it in a few moments, while waiting at stoplights in your car, or at your desk at the office.

1. Clarify your top priorities, both inner and outer.

2. Write these priorities on a piece of paper, on your computer, in your daily calendar, or on a note placed prominently on your

3. bathroom mirror. Keep them where you can see them frequently.

4. Once a day, reread them, evaluating where you are with each one and how you feel about it. Do this in a factual, detached way, and be careful not to use it as an opportunity to criticize or to be negative about anything you are doing.

5. For all the aspects of each priority you feel positive about, congratulate yourself sincerely, just the way you would like a friend to acknowledge you.

6. For all those aspects you feel unhappy about, consider what you could be doing differently or whether you need to re-evaluate that priority. For example, if you have a plan related to a priority and you're not carrying it out, you might ponder whether that priority is truly important to you, or whether you are stuck on it for other reasons that need to be handled, or whether life circumstances are just putting that priority on hold for a while. Megan, for example, did not know how long it would take her to find a suitable mate and then to become pregnant; she couldn't control that, but she could make sure she went one place per week (like a class) where she'd meet the caliber of man she wants for a partner. If she hadn't followed that plan, she would have evaluated why not. Perhaps she was experiencing relationship issues that still

needed to be worked out and some therapy was in order.

7. After you have reviewed your priorities and the current state of your plan, go about your daily tasks and don't worry about your priorities. You'll visit them again tomorrow, and in this way you'll keep them in balance.

If you follow these steps every day, you'll soon find that your priorities are becoming more solid and you are getting clearer on how to implement them—how to stay focused on them enough to create the life you want.

YOUR ROAD MAP TO SUCCESS

Once you have sorted out your priorities by doing the previous exercises, you can actually make a "road map" for yourself.

Creating a visual representation of what you want to achieve can do several things. First, the process of creating it will force you to be more specific and clear about what you want. Second, taking the time and energy to create it is a powerful signal to yourself that you are serious about accomplishing it. It sets an intention. Third, if you keep it where you can see it, it will be a powerful reminder of your intentions for your own life.

Your visual road map consists of two parts: (1) a picture of your destination and (2) your map of how to get there. The destination picture must come first because you cannot know how to get somewhere until you have a clear picture of where it is and what it looks like. This picture is developed from the information you accumulated in the previous exercises as you focused on your priorities and your dreams. Once it is completed, figuring out what steps you need to follow to create the results you want provides the details for creating your road map.

Road Map Exercise 1: Picturing Your Destination

It is not important for your finished picture to be artistic: only that it is an accurate representation of the goals you desire to accomplish. You may want to spend several sessions at this exercise, over several days or weeks, if necessary, to get your picture exactly the way you want it. Remember, this is a visual representation of your ideal life, and you will use it for the next several years to remind and motivate yourself, so treat it as the important project it is. When you look at your finished picture, you should be able to see each of your goals clearly represented.

Preparation

1. *Collect the materials necessary to make a collage you can write on: a large piece of paper and colored markers, pens, paints, pastels or other art materials; several magazines full of pictures and advertisements you can cut out; paste or a glue stick; and several photos of you and others in your life. If you enjoy drawing, you may want to dispense with the magazine pictures and draw your own. If you prefer, use computer art to do this. You can also add solid objects, pieces of cloth or jewelry, tokens and keepsakes that*

are meaningful to you. Keep in mind that colorful, graphic pictures are powerful subconscious stimulants, and the point of this exercise is to help you focus your subconscious on your goals and dreams. Choose a work space where you can spread out comfortably.

2. *Divide your paper into sections representing your personal life, your business or career, your family life, your friends and your free time.*

3. *Title each section, and think about what, if you designed your own life, you would want to create in that section.*

Creating Your Results Picture

4. *Begin with the personal life section and think about what activities represent the private, personal part of your life: including the images that symbolize you. Begin with a picture of you as you are, or as you would like to be (in a graduation gown, a wedding gown, thinner, successful, etc.—you can paste a small picture of your head or face on a magazine picture if you wish; or even dress up and take a selfie). Are there hobbies or talents that are important to you? What kinds of images make you feel good about yourself? What symbols would you use to represent yourself? What do you want to use to represent your physical health? Your happiness? Your determination? Choose one or two images to represent the various ways you identify yourself, such as the following:*

- *Gardening is one way you recharge yourself, so you use pictures of flower or vegetable gardens.*
- *Your spiritual or religious beliefs are central to your identity, so you include some symbols of those beliefs.*
- *You like to soak in the tub, so pictures of bubbles, soft towels and a luxurious bathtub provide satisfying images.*
- *Physical activity recharges you, so use pictures of a runner or sports champion.*
- *You identify yourself closely with your work, so you include picture of you in your best business suit.*
- *Your role as a mother is primary to you, so you include a photo of you holding a child.*
- *You like to be the center of attention, so you paste a photo of yourself into a picture of a crowd of admiring people that you cut from an ad.*
- *You love music, so you put some musical notes into the collage.*

5. *Look through the magazines for pictures of concrete items or goals that would complete the personal section of your road map, such as the following:*
   - *A suitable representation of your home: whether it is a dorm, a rented room, a house or an apartment.*

- *Other personal items that are important to you and represent your lifestyle, such as a car, sports equipment, clothing styles, etc.*

- *Pictures of travel or other vacation activities.*

- *Pictures to represent pets or other animals you have or desire to have.*

- *Personal growth goals, such as emotional growth, better physical health (through exercise, a healthy diet, etc.), spiritual or academic studies, and the like.*

- *Any other significant factors representing your personal life.*

6. *Arrange these pictures in the personal section of your collage in a way that suits you, or draw representations of the items that are important to you. Be sure your chosen picture of yourself is front and center in this personal section. Arrange and rearrange and adjust your collection of pictures until the final result pleases you.*

   Consider a background color appropriate to each section. For example, use your favorite color as the background for the personal section; metallic gold or green, to represent money for the business section; yellow, to represent sunshine for the free-time section; pink, to represent love for the friends or the family section. When you finish, the picture should be accurate enough so that anyone who looks at it (should you care to show it) will get an accurate representation of your own idea of who you are.

7. *Now complete the other sections of your results picture in a similar fashion. Each section will probably include some elements repeated from the personal section because you will be involved personally in each category. Use an image of your idealized self prominently in each section; either create a different version of your idealized self for each section, or use black-and-white or color photocopies of your original in each section.*

- **Your business or career,** *including pictures of your success, your desired career, your investments, business associates, business travel, degrees or diplomas, tools or products, your own business-building activities, etc. If your true vocation is not necessarily the way you make your living, include both your vocation and your livelihood in this section.*

- *Your family life, which can include your family of origin, your extended family, your future family and/or your family of friends. Even pets can be included here, if they feel like family elements to you. Arrange these various family members in relationship to each other, in the way you would like them to relate—you can draw lines to show how your family of origin and your future family will, ideally, be* connected, for example. Include favorite family occasions—past, present or future, such as evening gatherings, holidays, and reunions. If you want to work with your family, take vacations with them or live with them, represent that in the picture. If your family is widespread, and that is okay with you, include a map with various branches of the family represented and the desired visits or communication represented by small pictures of airplanes, cars, telephones, letters or computers. If you have lost beloved members of your family, you can also represent them here in symbolic ways. For example, if your grandmother has passed away, you can show things you once did together, or show her as an angel.

- **Your friends**, depending on how important they are to you, may be included in lieu of family, or in family, instead of in a section of their own. This section may also include representations of working together, free time spent together, shared hobbies or sports, etc.

- **Your free time**, because life is not all about work. Be sure to include your favorite hobbies, your leisure pursuits and pictures that symbolize fun to you.

Now that you're "getting the picture" you may be inspired to make more sections or change the format. Remember this is a picture of your life as you want it to *be, so put in whatever seems important to you. Don't hesitate to redesign your picture if you get better ideas about how it should look.*

When you have arranged your picture, stand back and take a look to see if it reflects your ideal life. If not, play with it some more; if it is, paste things down and place the collage where you can look at it often. This picture only needs to represent your future as you presently think it should be: you can alter your picture, add to it or make a new one as your goals grow and change.

Road Map Exercise 2: Making Your Road Map

Once you put the necessary time and energy into picturing your destination, you'll find that by focusing on specifics and details you have clarified your picture. Most of the women who have done this process in workshops and classes report that they feel very motivated, much clearer and energized by their vision. Take that energy and use it now to create your road map: a plan of action to get you to your destination.

1. *Use a separate piece of paper or artboard, and entitle the left side of the road map "Where I Am Now." Place sufficient symbols, words or numbers to indicate where you are now in all the areas outlined on your destination picture. For example:*

   - *In the area of business, perhaps you are just getting your degree, or maybe you are beginning to climb the ladder in your firm, or perhaps you have an idea for beginning a business of your own.*

- *In the area of family, you are still treated as a child by your*

- *parents, or you have left home and begun a new relationship with your birth family, or you have a partner and are building the foundation of your new family together.*

- *In the area of finances, you are saddled with college loans, or you're saving to buy a house of your own.*

2. *Title the right side of the paper or artboard "My Destination" and arrange symbols, words or numbers to indicate where you will be when you reach your goals. For example:*

   - *In the area of business, perhaps you want to be well-established, respected in your work, a senior partner in your firm or successful in your own business.*

   - *In the area of family, you want to achieve a warm and enjoy-able peer relationship with your parents and siblings, or be well-established in your own family and have a successful social and support system.*

   - *In the area of finances, you will be solidly established and secure in your own home with secure investments.*

3. *Divide the space between into columns. In those columns, develop the steps you'll need to accomplish to get from where you are now to your destination. For example:*

• *In the area of business, the steps might be (1) graduate from school; (2) do a job search; (3) develop career skills, experience and expertise; and (4) move up on your career ladder. (Each of these steps can be broken into smaller steps as you approach that segment of the road map and need to accomplish specific goals.)*

Use Your Road Map Daily

After completing your destination picture and road map, use them daily to remain focused on your goals and maintain your motivation. Keep them where you can review them frequently and change and update them as needed. You'll find that having a clear picture of your goals and aspirations in front of you will make it much easier to reach them.

All of your decisions from now on can be made in relationship to your road map. If you consider each of your subsequent decisions according to whether it will get you closer to your goal or not, your choices will become more clear and more direct.

Jodie discovered the power of business planning in her Junior Achievers class. By creating a clear and specific plan of action, and keeping her goals in mind, she realized that her community had a need and she successfully filled it with her restaurant-to-home delivery service. What she didn't realize was that all the other areas of her life could benefit from the same planning process. Because her business plan was the only one she had, and she was not quite prepared for her big success, business took over her whole life and she wound up feeling stressed and overwhelmed. By taking some time to make a picture of her destination and a road map, Jodie realized that she wanted more social and family contact in her life and more time to relax and have fun. She now follows her road map and is reorganizing her business to offer franchises so that she won't have to be so directly and constantly involved. She is beginning to plan for a personal life, too, including having a family of her own.

Using your destination picture and road map to set your priorities and to keep you focused will help you keep all the important areas of your life balanced and will help shape your future. Knowing where you want to go and how to get there will minimize your tendencies to worry and reduce your indecisiveness and confusion.

SACRIFICE: IS IT IMPORTANT?

This whole chapter, and even most of this book so far, may seem too focused on self-importance. Most of you probably care deeply about other people in your lives, especially your family, partners, and children, and don't want your life to be all about what you want and need. You want to care about others, and even to sacrifice for those you love. If you really try the ideas in this book, you'll find out they are completely compatible with having warm, loving relationships with others, even when, at times, those relationships become more important than the other goals in your life. That is one reason for the emphasis here on achieving a balance in many ways, including between your own wants and those of others. Becoming successful at the cost of not having time for close relationships is, as Jodie found, too high a price to pay. For that reason, your road map and destination picture include sections about family and friends.

FUTURE GOOD VERSUS PRESENT HAPPINESS

There are things you need to sacrifice today in order to have your plan in place for tomorrow.

> *Kisha started on welfare with two small children and no education, so she had to work extra hard to get ahead. Once she decided to make a better life for herself and her children, she created a clear picture of her destination and she was determined to reach her goals. In the next few years, she sacrificed a lot. She rarely went out because she needed to study and to take care of her children and she didn't have enough money to afford babysitters. Though her school provided low-cost daycare, she had no extra funds. Later on, you'll see how Kisha used a "village" or support system to make her life a bit more workable, but for about five years she had no*

luxuries and no extravagances. By making that sacrifice in the beginning of her road map, Kisha was able to reach a destination where she and her children are financially secure and comfortable. By postponing the natural wishes of a young woman to own pretty things and to have fun, Kisha was able to reach her goals more quickly and get herself to where she wanted to be.

There are a number of future goals that you may consider worthy of sacrifice:

• Postponing vacations or doing inexpensive things like camping or day trips in order to save for a down payment on a house.

• Putting your career goals on a slower track in order to be a mother first.

• Finishing your education before getting married.

• Waiting until your business is well-established before having a baby.

• Postponing career goals, education or marriage to care for a seriously ill or aging family member.

• Staying at a job you don't really like in order to finance your education, a new house or a business venture.

• Forgoing a new car purchase in order to build up your savings or retirement account.

• Taking a second job to pay off accumulated bills.

- Investing the time and energy to lose weight or to perfect a hobby to boost your self-esteem.

- Changing your schedule to make time for meditation in order to reduce stress or improve your health.

In appropriate circumstances, any of these sacrifices, whether large or small, can be a good investment in your final destination. Even though your future plans may seem postponed or put off in order to create a better foundation or to devote time to removing an obstacle or achieving another more urgent goal, in the long run your destination will be more complete and satisfying if you take the extra time to do what is most important to you.

Sharon's goal was to utilize her MBA in a fast-track career, but when she discovered that the jobs in her hometown were not plentiful, she had to make a decision. By setting priorities, she realized that her hometown environment, including family and friends, was even more important to her than her career goals, so she decided to put her career on a slower track in order to keep the quality of her life and to support her emotional well-being and personal values. Sharon found that an excellent career was still available but would take a few years longer to achieve in her smaller city. **Kim**'s destination picture, on the other hand, made it very clear to her that her family's well-intentioned pressure was threatening to push her onto a career track in medicine that she was not sure she wanted. Once she got some help in viewing the future from her own desires, rather than from fears of disappointing the people who loved and supported her, she was easily able to find a medical career (pediatrics) that would both satisfy her personal wants and also make her family happy and proud.

Deciding to evaluate your future priorities and making a road map to follow give you the best possibility of creating a future that is compatible with who you are and your life circumstances.

4
Who Loves Ya, Baby?
Decide to Make the Most of Who You Are

***

There are two ways of spreading light: to be the candle or the mirror that reflects it.

—Edith Wharton

***

You are already a marvelous package of talents, skills, experience and personality traits. The problem is that many women are far too self-critical and self-deprecating, and if you treat yourself that way you'll have a difficult time evaluating yourself objectively. Learning to think positively about who you are, and thereby making the best of each of your traits and talents, will enable you to operate at your most powerful and to be truly satisfied with the results.

THE POWER OF KNOWING YOURSELF

The popular book by John Gray, *Men Are from Mars, Women Are from Venus,* uses the metaphor of people growing up on different planets to illustrate how differently men and women perceive and react to stimuli and events. Actually, as individuals we have many more differences than those connected to gender. Even when comparing women, it often seems as if each of us grew up on a distinct planet with a completely unique approach to life. Our accumulated experiences and our individual traits combine to make us different. You may not even feel that other members of your own family are much like you. These differences can be problems in some ways, but the ways in which you are different from others can also be your greatest assets.

Taking stock of your talents, traits and characteristics is fundamentally important to using who you are to the fullest. You may have always thought you were too quiet or too talkative, too aggressive or too passive: but what happens if you reevaluate "too quiet" to mean that you're a good listener, or "too talkative" to mean you are an excellent communicator? Traits you evaluate as too aggressive can turn out to be leadership qualities, and "too passive" traits can mean you're an excellent support or follow-up person. Thinking of all the possibilities of human personality characteristics as distinct colors in a palette makes it possible to realize that each of the colors can be useful in the appropriate circumstance. Becoming aware and learning about yourself by increasing your ability to see new options and solutions increases your success and effectiveness, giving you the confidence you need to succeed and the accurate self-evaluation you need to make appropriate decisions and succeed.

So how do you discover the special colors of your own personal palette?

You probably think of yourself in several roles, such as daughter, student, employee, friend, sister, lover, perhaps mother or, on a date, even a femme fatale. None of us is just one person. At one time, hearing "voices in your head" was thought to mean you were crazy, but several decades ago many modes of psychotherapy (including psychosynthesis, transactional analysis, Gestalt and Jungian therapy) recognized that inner voices are normal and that everyone has some kind of mental commentary going on most of the time. These therapies began to focus on these voices of our minds and developed methods for dialogue that creates inner harmony by resolving the conflicting ideas into cooperating parts of a mental "team." Many techniques have been suggested to help people who want to know themselves better to get in touch with these personae, including hypnosis, writing with your non-dominant hand, journaling and various internal dialogues, all of which are helpful.

Another effective tool you can use is your mirror. Mirrors provide a simple way to become aware of yourself and to learn to use all your various characteristics to maximize your success and happiness. "Mirror work is very powerful," writes Louise Hay in *You Can Heal Your Life*. "To look yourself straight in the eye and make a positive declaration about yourself is, in my opinion, the quickest way to get results." "To cultivate a friendship with myself I find that I need to take time each day [in front of a mirror] to sit with myself," writes Carol Putnam in "My Selves in the Mirror." "I continue to make new acquaintances of a multitude of sub-personalities... I recognize myself as...the Unlovable Child, the Valedictorian, the Advocate, the Helper, the Rebel, the New Age Critic... and Company. From this place... I can observe, direct and harmonize my mental, physical and emotional processes... I can welcome home all the parts of me that I exiled long ago."

Exercise: Your Selves in the Mirror

To do your own mirror work, follow these steps:

1. **Choose a mirror.** *Get comfortable in a private place. In the beginning, a small hand mirror for the face only, is best. Later, as you become more adept, you can use a bigger mirror if you like.*

2. **Greet yourself.** *Look at your eyes in the mirror. Call yourself by name, and tell yourself hello the same way you would to a good friend. If talking to yourself in this way feels strange, allow yourself some time to get comfortable.*

3. **Listen to your inner selves.** *Sit quietly, close your eyes to help you concentrate and listen to your inner self. Chances are you will become aware of several "voices" that are commenting in your mind. At first, you may hear nothing, or a confusing babble of several inner voices talking at once, but if you allow some time and wait patiently, what they say will begin to become*

clear. You may have inner "voices" saying: "I want to take the new job. I need a change." or "I'm scared. Everything will be new and unpredictable." or "I'd better stay where I am. I could fail." or "I don't want to make this decision myself." At this point, you will probably hear some negative inner voices. Listen to what they say, then counteract them in the same way you handled your anxieties in the Worrier's Guidelines in Chapter 1, by responding to them with anxiety alleviating statements or actions. Becoming aware of these negative voices may be uncomfortable, but it will give you a chance to see what your anxieties are about and to soothe them.

You may only get as far as this step the first few times you do this exercise. If so, use the Worrier's Guidelines until the inner negative voices calm down, then say "thank you" to yourself in the mirror and end the exercise for the day. When this step becomes easier, go on to step 4.

4. **Identify your aspects**. *When you have spent some time with yourself, your inner voices will begin to differentiate and feel like individual personality characteristics or attitudes such as grown-up and child. (Grown-up: "You have to get some work done." Child: "I want to play.") But some of my clients have called theirs Dreamer and Pragmatist. (Dreamer: "Wouldn't it be nice if we won the lottery and didn't have to*

work?" Pragmatist: "The odds are terrible. We'd be better off saving the money.") Others call theirs Male and Female, Procrastinator and Nagger. When you have distinguished two or more voices, give each one a name to differentiate them. The names can be people's names (Joe, Mary) or descriptive, like those above. One of my clients has two main arguing voices she calls Rebel and Visionary. Another woman has a whole crowd, with whimsical names such as Hysterical Harriet, Angry Amy, Pleasing Pauline, Critical Carl, Depressed Debra and Rusty Resistance.

5. **Get acquainted with your inner selves.** *Give each one a turn to talk, and listen to their points of view. Becoming aware of what your internal selves are saying will give you insight into all your talents, dreams and wishes. As you get more comfortable, you'll find you can ask these imaginary parts of yourself questions and have discussions with them. Especially whenever you are un decided, or "of two minds" about a decision, discussing all the aspects of the situation with your inner selves will help clarify your confusion. (For example, Practical Self: "This is a good job, with good benefits, take it." Child Self: "I don't like the boss man. He isn't very nice.")*

6. **If you get confused, write it down.** *If your inner selves have too many differences over a particular issue, it may be difficult to keep them*

separate, so if doing this exercise solely in your imagination feels too difficult, write out the different points of view on paper, where you can become aware of them in an orderly fashion. Make a column or a page for each self, and briefly write out that voice's opinion on the issue in question, until the issues are clear and you can work out a solution.

7. **Reach agreement**. *Continue the session until you reach an acceptable agreement that satisfies all parts of yourself.*

8. **Repeat to become proficient.** *By doing this exercise several times, you will become more comfortable with your inner selves, their strengths and weaknesses, and even when you become aware of several different attitudes and opinions, you'll know how to handle them better and thereby be more in charge. Each time you repeat these steps, you will have an easier time identifying and understanding all the various aspects of yourself, including those aspects you were previously unaware of. Soon you will be able to "negotiate" internal problems very quickly, eliminate the internal confusion and think much more clearly.*

Follow-Up Exercise: Daily Routine

Once you're comfortable and familiar with all the parts of your inner self, try using your new self-

awareness to create a daily routine, either in the morning or the evening.

Morning Routine: *Make some agreements with yourself to make your day fun, to accomplish something, to reward yourself for work well done, or to give yourself some rest and relaxation. Wish yourself a happy day.*

Evening Routine: *Review your day in reverse order of events and be sure to praise and thank yourself for everything you accomplished during the day. Appreciate yourself for getting up in the morning, for doing your work, for caring for yourself. Praise yourself for work well done, for new ideas, for kindnesses to yourself and others. If there was a problem in your day, give some thought to how to correct it or how to do it differently next time without criticizing yourself. When you finish your review, close a mental door on it and don't allow yourself to think about it anymore that evening.*

Sharon *was used to second-guessing herself. No matter what decisions she made, she worried that it was the wrong one. "After I learned to review my day every evening and plan my day every morning, I realized that I could make good decisions. I had just never taken the time to think it all through before. I was too used to asking someone else for advice." Sharon found that she gradually gained more confidence in her decisions. And her decisions, being so much more carefully considered and monitored on a daily basis, became more reliable as a result. Sharon's confidence grew, and she was able to create the life she always wanted.*

MOTIVATION AND HOW TO CREATE IT

Many women complain of a lack of motivation from not being motivated enough on the job, to not being able to diet, get work done, quit smoking, or follow through on their goals and decisions. They desire to achieve both positive and negative motivations: positive motivations toward doing or being something and negative motivations toward not doing something.

Almost invariably, the method they have tried before unsuccessfully has been to beat themselves into it. This happens through a negative inner dialogue, such as: "You lazy person. You'll never get anywhere." or "You have to do this whether you like it or not." or "No one will ever love you until you do." At times, they have tried bribing or persuading themselves, which works for a while but fails sooner or later. Alternatively, they have gotten other people to make decisions for them, such as a motivational group, a hypnotist, a parent or parent substitute who will insist that they behave.

This third option often works quite well for some women for a long time. However, the nature of this persuasion is to overpower your natural process. Sooner or later, whether you push yourself with internal criticism or enlist someone else to do it, you'll eventually feel oppressed and rebellious. Motivation through intimidation and pressure eventually results in paralysis and procrastination.

In my experience, the only kind of motivation that works permanently grows out of celebration and appreciation. I like to state it in equation: *celebration + appreciation = motivation.*

This means when you find a way to appreciate yourself for what you've already accomplished and to celebrate your previous successes, you will find you are naturally motivated to accomplish more. No struggle, no hassle: you accomplish out of the pure joy of success! To illustrate this concept, consider two possible employers: the "bad boss" and the "good boss."

The Bad Boss

- Operates through intimidation and criticism.

- Always complains, never praises (you only know you're doing okay because the boss says nothing).

- Gets nasty if you make a mistake.

- Humiliates you in front of others.

- Never thinks you've done enough.

- Assumes you are lazy and dishonest.

- Changes the rules arbitrarily.

- Is never satisfied or pleased.

The Good Boss

- Praises frequently.

- Always lets you know when you're doing well.

- Asks you what you need whenever you've made a mistake.

- Is very helpful.

- Is concerned about your well-being as well as your productivity.

- Assumes you want to do a good job.

- Helps you feel like part of the team.

- Treats you as a valued human being.

- Is clear about the duties expected of you.

Both of these bosses have the same goal: to get the job done. However, there is a big difference in the success of their individual management styles.

What would your reaction be to working with each of these bosses? If you worked for the bad boss, you would probably work in an atmosphere of tension and anger. You'd work only to keep the boss off your back and be tempted to goof off whenever he/she is not around. You would not be your most efficient because you'd be stressed and resentful.

If you were working for this boss, how would you feel? Would you go to work happily each day? Would you volunteer for extra work? Would you look forward to each new assignment? Probably not. In short, you would not feel highly motivated, would you?

On the other hand, working for the good boss would tend to make you care about your productivity and your job. You'd take pride in your accomplishments, be eager to learn more and accomplish more. Even in such a boss's absence you would work well, be motivated, and feel gratified and appreciated. Anything your boss asks would be met with a cooperative response.

How would you feel? Would you feel eager to please this boss? Would you look forward to his/her reaction to your latest work? Would you be willing to help out if extra work were necessary? Most likely, you would—you would feel enthusiastic and motivated, looking forward to work each day.

Which boss would you rather work for?

In being in charge of your own life, you become your own boss and you have a choice about which kind of boss you want to be to yourself. To become the good boss to yourself you must treat yourself with kindness and understanding, be very generous with praise and gentle with corrections. Then you will accomplish your goals with a sense of pride and achievement, and a great deal of pleasure. You will feel motivated and wonder why you never realized how easy it was.

All of this can be accomplished through the two "magic motivators": celebration and appreciation. Most of us know how to appreciate others. However, when it comes to ourselves we feel embarrassed and uncomfortable if we are too generous with praise.

Years of being told not to brag or be cocky when we were young have taken their toll, and self-appreciation comes awkwardly. However, if motivation is a desirable trait, self-appreciation becomes necessary and desirable, too. The good news is that you can learn it.

GUIDELINES FOR LEARNING APPRECIATION

To become proficient in self-appreciation, try the following suggestions:

- Buy small gold-foil star stickers (just like in grade school) and award them to yourself for jobs well done or any achievements you want to celebrate. Pasting the stars on a calendar daily can be very effective. Other kinds of stickers are readily available. Rita rewarded herself for sticking to her weight loss program with small stickers representing jelly beans, chocolates and ice cream cones! She got her dessert in praise instead of calories.

- Remember back to what felt like a celebration in your childhood. Kim was told never to make noise because her grandmother was ill. However, she was allowed to play the piano as loud as she wanted to when she practiced. To this day, playing the piano feels like a celebration and a chance for her to sound off. Kisha had few luxuries in her childhood, but she remembers the feeling of the bubble baths her mother used to give her for a treat. It still feels special to her to soak in a hot tub of fragrant bubbles.

- Use elements of your favorite early birthday parties or holiday outings that were special. If Mom always cooked a turkey for a big occasion, or set the table with the best china, those ingredients can indicate celebration and accomplishment.

- Fresh flowers say how much you appreciate yourself and can do a lot toward making you happier any day.

- A trashy romance novel can be a great reward/celebration for reading your required technical books.

- Celebrate a cherished friendship with an impromptu lunch-time picnic and a balloon.

By celebrating your accomplishments, however small, you will create motivation to accomplish more. Get creative with your celebrations. Above all, have fun.

BE YOUR OWN BOSS

If you find yourself around someone who takes command and tells you what you should be doing or offers unsolicited comments about how you are doing things wrong, or otherwise appoints him/herself as the boss in your life, you may find your newly created motivation flagging. Remember, you can mentally fire this person as your boss. It's your life, and you are following your own carefully considered road map. Anytime you have to "fire" a bad boss, you may need to remind yourself how much you have accomplished without that kind of help. Celebrate your independence, your spirit, your willingness to be responsible for yourself.

It is also possible to set up informative books, articles, television authorities, gurus and the like as your boss: in which case you will again find your rebellion rising and your motivation flagging. These informational aids can be useful: but only if you keep them in perspective.

Remember, the boss gets information about how to run things, gets educated, goes for help when necessary, but the boss is in charge. The boss's information is there for your use, but no outside expert (not even a therapist) can know if the information is right for you. By being your own internal boss, you will use the information wisely and judiciously, rejecting whatever there is that does not suit your style or personality or move you closer to your chosen destination. You will use it to support and further your goals and to aid in the celebration of your accomplishments.

Whenever you find your motivation flagging, look around for how you are doing at being your boss. Are you using a motivational, supportive style? Have you let someone else take over your authority? Is there some appreciation you need?

Take a few minutes with yourself every day just for appreciation. It's easy, fun and very effective. Imagine living every day energized and motivated!

YOUR SOCIAL SKILLS

Reaching your chosen destination requires that you get along with other people. This category includes, among other skills, behavior and manners, communication skills, and the ability to empathize.

Socially acceptable behavior and manners vary with circumstances and the situation and people involved. For example, if you want to succeed as a high-ranking politician or a diplomat, you must be quite skilled at protocol and know appropriate dress and behavior for many situations, even the mores of other cultures. On the other hand, if you want to work with small children, your behavior can be a lot more casual and relaxed. Emotional empathy and patience are valuable skills if you're dealing with children.

In this way, the road map decisions dictate the amount of social skillfulness we will require to succeed. Social adeptness can make a huge difference in how successful you are in your work, with friends and associates, and at home.

"We send emotional signals in every encounter," writes Daniel Goleman in his groundbreaking book, *Emotional Intelligence,* "and those signals affect those we are with. The more adroit we are socially, the better we control the signals we send: the reserve of polite society is, after all, simply a means to ensure that no disturbing emotional leakage will unsettle the encounter... Emotional intelligence includes managing this exchange: 'popular' and 'charming' are terms we use for people whom we like to be with because their emotional skills make us feel good. People who are able to help others soothe their feelings have an especially valued social commodity; they are the souls others turn to when in greatest emotional need. We are all part of each other's tool kit for emotional exchange, for better or for worse."

While Goleman's book can help educate you about emotional intelligence, Judith Martin's very readable books give practical advice for making your way in the world smoothly, with self-confidence, because you know the proper social forms.

"If you aim for a position in which you never need people to vote for you, to support your policies, to do any work for you, to buy tickets to your shows, to defend your life and your property, to make you look good in the eyes of your own superiors or constituents, to treat you with respect, to come to your aid when you need it, to admire you, to refrain from ridiculing you, to abstain from plotting ways of getting you out of your position, to support you in rising even further, or to shed a tear when you are dead," writes Judith Martin in *Miss Manners' Guide for the Turn-of the-Millennium*, "then you can probably trample on the feelings of others in relative safety."

> *Kisha, who was raised in an atmosphere of poverty and lack of education, found she had trouble understanding how to behave in social situations in school and, later, in work. She found that reading books on social and business etiquette helped her understand the behavior of the people around her and to fit in more comfortably.*
>
> *Kim, whose family was from another culture, found that classes and books about business and social etiquette helped her sort out her cultural confusion. As a medical student, her understanding of her native cultural rules was very helpful when dealing with the ethnic mix of patients in the hospital, and she often advised other students in this regard.*

Kim and Kisha both discovered that there are ethnic, social and educational differences that can contribute to social confusion, and make it difficult to understand others.

"Each person's life is lived as a series of conversations," writes sociolinguist Deborah Tannen in her bestselling book, *You Just Don't Understand: Women and Men in Conversation.* "People have different conversational styles. So, when speakers from different parts of the country, or of different ethnic or class backgrounds, talk to each other, it is likely that their words will not be understood exactly as they were meant."

But, as both Kim and Kisha learned, spending time learning about the social mores of the types of people they wanted to socialize with (in this case, professional and business people) helped them to communicate more effectively, and send social signals others understood.

SOOTHING, REASSURING AND RELAXING YOURSELF

The final advantage of knowing who you are is knowing how to pamper and comfort yourself when you're stressed or tired. Use what you have learned about your celebration style to develop a style for recharging and relaxing. What makes you most comfortable? What soothes you? What helps you recharge? It can be anything from a bubble bath, a yoga session, or your favorite music to a long walk in the country, a phone conversation with your best friend, or a nap. Make a list of your favorite "personal rechargers." Make sure the list includes simple things you can do cheaply (such as relax with a cup of tea and read a favorite book) to things that are very special (such as spend a night at a bed and breakfast or have a massage and a facial). Keep the list where you can refer to it whenever you feel in need of a recharge, and make use of it often. Marie finds music to be the most soothing and recharging experience in her life. When she wants to recharge, she listens to her favorite opera arias on CD or sings her favorites as a form of meditation.

MAKING YOUR DREAMS A REALITY

By becoming acquainted with who you are, you can tailor all your decisions precisely to fit your life. By following your road map, keeping your chosen destination in mind, learning to motivate yourself through celebration and appreciation and recharging yourself, you can keep your energy high and follow through on the decisions you make.

Using effective communication will help you enlist others to join in your projects and will make your family life and friendships run smoothly. With these tools, you can implement all of your decisions and make your dreams come true.

The self you learn to recognize today is already changing: life experience, contact with others, and learning and growing change who we are constantly. By making the exercises in this chapter part of your daily life, you can keep up with your changing abilities and know-how, make self-awareness a lifelong, creative process, and continue to use what you know about yourself to set your priorities. Through appreciation and celebration, you can keep yourself continually motivated, gently yet effectively, until you complete your road map to success.

5
Go for the Goals:
Decide to Get the Education and
Training You Need

***

*If you think you can, you can. And if
you think you can't, you're right.*

—Mary Kay Ash

***

Wherever your destination picture and your road map lead you, the proper education will make your journey easier and your success more assured. But what kind of education is the right education? Today, most of us think of education as a college degree, but there are many kinds. The path you choose to follow may indeed require college, or it may lead you to another type of education.

THE NEW TECHNOLOGY:
WHAT DO YOU NEED TO KNOW?

Today we live in a highly specialized society, and life is getting more and more complex. When your grandparents were your age, their house contained few items that were too complicated to understand or fix with simple tools and techniques. Today, our homes are filled with appliances and machinery that take vast amounts of training to understand. How many of us can repair our own television, microwave oven, computer, tablet or smart phone, not to mention stereo, clock radio, DVD player, washer, dryer, dishwasher, video camera, fax machine, copier, automatic heating thermostat or air conditioner? This same complexity exists everywhere we go, including work.

Never before have human beings had so much electronic assistance, and so much confusion about it. Our computers, smart phones, Bluetooth devices, TVs and other equipment now become obsolete often before they're paid off. The speed with which things change can be very intimidating, and each new piece of equipment requires learning. A new innovation in technology has changed entire industries (like book publishing) overnight.

No matter what your goals and aspirations, learning to use computers and the Internet is essential. It won't be long before a person's knowledge of computers, electronics, software, programming and the Internet will divide society into "haves" (those who know how to use the technology) and "have nots" (those who don't). Not knowing how to use smart devices and the Internet will soon be tantamount to being illiterate, dooming people to low-paying jobs.

Whether you're a parent who wants to ask other people on the Internet about discipline or childhood illnesses, a high-tech computer programmer, a customer in a bank or library, or a store clerk, you'll find that Web-streaming and smart devices have become a basic tool for everyone today. Computers and the Internet are also tools you can use to get an education.

Are you using too much or too little technology in your life? If you came of age before the Millennium, computers and other technology remain a mystery. Even knowing about technology and how to use it in a specific situation (for example, word processing on a computer at your job) does not necessarily mean you understand all the ways it can and should be used in your life.

RESISTANCE

Many women resist the changes involved in bringing new technology into their lives. Men still tend to be more computer-savvy than many women. Many video games and Web sites are male-oriented (although there is a rising market in women-oriented games and CD-ROMs). Yet, even though women tend to be more represented on the Internet for shopping, it is a treasure trove of information and well worth overcoming any resistance you have toward it.

Resistance to new information and equipment is usually the result of unfamiliarity. New technology can be intimidating: with an abundance of computer peripherals, software, and applications, there is a lot to learn. Until you learn it, the newness can be overwhelming.

Marie *loves classical music and musical instruments with histories going back hundreds of years. To her, computers and technology were unnecessary and uncomfortable. "I thought of electronic music as a threat, which was putting classically trained musicians out of business," said Marie, "but while I was getting my music degree and teacher's certification, I discovered how much musical research could be conducted on the Internet, and how much fun children could have learning music on electronic keyboards. When I became familiar with what technology could do, I realized how useful it could be."*

Computer programs and MIDI (Musical Instrument Digital Interface) technology enabled Marie to bypass the tedious work of writing out musical arrangements for her choir: she could simply play the arrangement on a keyboard connected to her computer, and the MIDI software would print out whatever was played on the keyboard. While technology was changing the music business, it was creating more new jobs for musicians (even classically trained ones) than it was eliminating. Electronic keyboards, rhythm synthesizers, mixing boards, the new digital recording capabilities, YouTube and other online videos, and even virtual reality make it possible for musicians and groups to share their music more easily and widely than ever before. Through the Internet, Marie is able to connect with musicians and music schools in Europe and around the world, to arrange exchange programs, and to set up concert tours so she can spend her summer on the Continent.

GETTING AND STAYING CURRENT

If technology intimidates you, there are many ways you can bring yourself up-to-date. The two ways most people get involved in computers and the Internet is through online information, classes or with the help of friends. There are office supply and copy shops in every small town and cafés which have Wi-Fi and libraries everywhere have free computer access. If you are in school or employed, find someone else who knows how to operate the more technical equipment and apps and ask for help or instruction. Neighbors, fellow students, business colleagues, friends and family members who know technology are usually flattered to be asked and happy to help. **Kisha** was very intimidated by computers and software, but when she got into her training school she found several other young women, some of them with similar histories, who all helped each other with assignments. The group support really helped Kisha relax and learn.

Even if you are the local technology whiz, it's essential to stay up-to-date. If you're employed in a career that can or does use technology, your employer will often pay for relevant workshops and classes. If your company doesn't already offer to assist you in your education, find some classes you'd like to take and make a proposal to your boss: you may find that the company is happy to help you because you become a more valuable employee. If you're self-employed, continuing education in your field is a legitimate business deduction.

***Megan's** new field, family law, is rapidly changing. Technology issues such as in vitro fertilization, surrogate parents, DNA evidence, and sperm banks require constant updating of the law. Megan's firm is happy to pay for information seminars.*

*In medical school, **Kim** was bombarded with new technology. MRIs and CAT scans, microscopic video cameras, laser surgery, Gamma knives. Tele-medicine and other high-tech equipment constantly create new career categories.*

Whatever the technology involved in your job, it's bound to be changing and expanding at a very rapid rate. The woman who can keep up with technology will have the edge. To keep up-to-date, use the technology. The Internet and the World Wide Web are the most up-to-date sources for information about technological advances. Learn to use them, and take the time to search out the sites, forums and chats that pertain to your career and your life.

Professional and trade journals, union magazines, seminars, conferences and expos are excellent sources of the newest information about your particular field. Most companies and employers will pay for all or part of the cost.

*To maintain her license as a substance abuse counselor **Robin** needs to earn education hours each year. When she looked for classes, she was delighted to find some in the business end of counseling, computers and insurance billing* *would qualify. She also found seminars in therapy techniques she wanted to learn. Joining professional organizations for women and counselors provided mentoring and support.*

*On the Internet, **Rita** got support from other working moms, including advice, how-to hints, emotional support, referrals to Web sites, and a safe place to vent frustrations. She also used work skills on her home computer and in apps to balance her checkbook and help the school PTA keep a mailing list and newsletter.*

THE RIGHT EDUCATIONAL PATH

No matter what your age or education, further study may turn out to be a good idea for you. If you have a clear, detailed picture of your destination and you've carefully created your road map to include specific directions and steps to take, you may already know the kind of education you need to get from where you are to where you want to be.

DEGREE OR NO DEGREE: THE REAL QUESTION

A traditional college education is not always the right way to go for what you want to accomplish. There are many technically oriented educations, such as nursing school or real estate school, which give you the specifics you need to do a particular kind of work. Many employers will pay for education that fits certain criteria related to your job.

Professional organizations, such as the American Association of Marriage and Family Therapists (www.aamft.org) and the American Society of Journalists and Authors (www.asja.org) offer classes and training for their members, scholarships for students majoring in their fields, and the mentoring benefits of peer-to-peer contact with professionals in the field.

The key to figuring out what kind of education and/or training you need is knowing your goals and the educational standards for those goals.

*At first, **Kim**'s choices seemed simple. Her family wanted her to be a doctor, so she got her pre-med degree. But applying to medical schools was a shock. So many choices to make! Deciding now to focus on internal medicine, psychiatry, oncology, geriatrics, emergency medicine, pediatrics, surgery, obstetrics and gynecology, or other specializations would affect which teaching hospitals, fellowships, and residencies would accept her later on. Kim was completely overwhelmed, and questioned whether medicine was the right career choice. While completing her road map she decided she needed a mentor's help. She asked her HMO personal physician, who invited her to a professional meeting. There, she met several other doctors, who invited her to visit their hospitals, surgeries, birthing centers and emergency rooms. She discovered she liked either obstetrics or pediatrics, which focused her on the teaching hospitals with the best pediatric departments, and the most respected pediatric medicine schools.*

Other careers require different kinds of education.

Kisha could not afford a college education, so she found a government training program which trained her as a computer operator and provided child care. Once trained, she got a job with a salary which was enough to support herself and her children. "Now that the kids are in school," Kisha says, "I want to train as a computer programmer." Her office pays for part of her education, which will raise her earning power. Kisha knows rapid changes in computer programs will require continuous reeducation, and her salary can keep rising.

Education can also give you more freedom and flexibility in your work.

Rita enjoyed her full-time office job, but found it took her away from her family too much, so she decided to study tax accounting, and be self-employed. Then, she and her insurance-agent husband set up an office in their home. Now they both work from home, and their flexible hours mean more family time.

EDUCATION BY DEGREES

There are many professions, such as nursing, counseling and teaching, for which you can obtain a lesser degree, work for a time and slowly add more education. For example, with a two-year degree, you can become a licensed vocational nurse and begin working, then get your bachelor's degree to become a registered nurse, and with further education become a nurse practitioner or a nursing supervisor or a nursing instructor. These tiers of learning and education can enable you to begin earning quickly in your chosen field, and then to move up, with some of your education credits often subsidized by your workplace. By arranging your education or training in tiers, you can work your way up the pay scale as you complete each phase of your studies.

DISCOVER THE NEW SCHOOLS

A relatively new phenomenon, there are many schools currently designed for adults who are working. A number of these schools are fully accredited and often provide an excellent education. Their programs are designed to meet whatever licensing requirements or professional standards a field requires, and they include such innovative features as the following:

Life-experience credits: If you have been working for a number of years (including as a housewife and mother) and then go back to school, some colleges will give you college credits for your years of experience. By documenting your life experiences in accordance with the rules of the school, you can obtain credit for completing courses. This can save you as much as a year of school.

Self-study courses: In many colleges, it is possible to set up your own course outline, workshops, experiments, reading and practical experiences to learn the subject matter, and a lot of courses are online. You must document what you learn in a way that meets the requirements of the course to earn full credit. In this way, you can set up your curriculum so that you learn exactly what you want to learn, completely on your own, without attending scheduled classes. Through online college classes, you may even be able to get a very low-cost or free education, entirely online.

Online courses: There are a number of reputable online courses, and if you are interested in a field in which one of these is offered, you can do the work at home, on your own time. These option allow you to work at your own pace and at hours convenient for you (for example, at night, after the children are asleep). This is an excellent, affordable way to learn technical details about your chosen field. Certificates for completing such courses are often accepted by universities and employers. Some employers will even pay part or all of your tuition.

Mentor programs: Many of these education programs offer mentoring, in which a recognized expert in the field (sometimes someone of your choice) is paid (through your tuition) to meet with you and teach you directly. Upon documenting what you learn, you receive credit as though you have attended a class. Under this system, it's often also possible to attend workshops in your field and get academic credit for them.

Evenings and weekends: To help you integrate your schooling and your work schedule, some programs offer classes on evenings and weekends. For example, you might meet with a core study group one or two nights a week and one weekend a month.

With such flexible options, alternative education can make it possible for you to earn a degree in your field while working full time, and to earn it much faster than you would in a traditional school. These courses of study are usually more expensive than most state or community college classes, but they often offer payment plans and financial aid.

You also can get the first two years of your college degree at a two-year community college or online, which is usually a very inexpensive option, and transfer to a bigger, more prestigious school for the last two years. That way you would get a four-year degree from the more expensive college or university for a lot less money.

The Internet and your local library are great sources of education. If you aspire to certain careers, such as medical doctor, nurse-midwife, electronics engineer or pilot, military service is an often overlooked avenue.

EDUCATION AND NETWORKING

As Kim discovered, getting connected with the proper people can be an education in itself. This process works in two ways. First, while getting your education in college, university, training school, or various workshops and clinics, you'll meet other people in your field, including the instructors, and each of these people can be a resource for you. Second, if you contact people who work in your desired career, either by interviewing them, or by attending meetings of professional organizations, or through people you already know, you can meet experts who can give you information from inside the career. It is well-known that for certain careers, such as politics, law, medicine, the arts, movies and drama, the prestigious universities are powerful partly because by going there you'll make connections you can draw on all your life.

Today, there are enough women in positions of power that the more prestigious women's universities and colleges are also powerful sources of networks. If knowing well-connected people is important to your chosen career, your choice of educational institution can make a big difference.

As you begin to meet people who are successful in your chosen area, there are several techniques you can use to strengthen the connections and build your network. There are ways to identify the people who are most important to know and those you can learn from, as well as specific techniques you can use to enlarge and strengthen your network and support systems. These techniques and guidelines are found in chapter 8, "It Takes a Village."

Because an educational setting will immerse you in a rich mixture of people who have talent and expertise in the very area of your focus (including teachers, professors, other students and visiting experts) it is the perfect opportunity to begin building a network that will last a lifetime.

YOU NEEDN'T BE A GENIUS

We tend to think of education as related to IQ and test scores, but there are many kinds of learning. If you've done a good job of identifying who you are and have chosen your goal appropriately, you can draw on the talent and abilities you have. You can get the education or training you need, even if you're a working mom from a disadvantaged background like Kisha. Don't defeat yourself by thinking education or training is too difficult for you.

There are several types of nonacademic education that are very valuable, including mentoring, apprenticeship, life and job experience, and technical training.

Mentoring: Learning from an expert in your field can be an excellent way to acquire a personalized, specialized education. In fact, in some fields (such as professional animal training, certain arts and some mechanical repair skills) there may be no other way to learn other than having a working expert in the field teach you as you work together. This can be arranged in an official way, where you make a clear arrangement with your mentor, or it can happen informally. Mentors can also be family members. In acting families, we often see the result of mentoring, as in the Fonda family, where Henry Fonda was the first member of his family to become an actor, and his children and their children are following in his footsteps.

Apprenticeship: An apprenticeship is a more formal type of mentoring and usually occurs within trade unions. For example, if you'd like to be a professional electrician, you join the electrician's union as an apprentice, and through training, union-sponsored classes, and work experience you work up through journeyman and eventually to master. Apprentices hip has a long, respected history in the world of fine arts, and many training programs in the arts, such as ballet schools, are actually apprentice programs in which you study and work in your field, working your way up as you learn and acquire expertise.

Job Experience: On-the-job experience can be a great teacher also. Many careers are learned mostly within the work setting. Sometimes it is very helpful to document what you have learned (by getting life-experience college credit, for example) so that your hard-won expertise is recognized by others.

Technical Training: There are also technical trade schools that tailor their programs around a specific technical skill, such as automotive mechanics school, dental technician school, fashion design school or a restaurant management school. These schools offer very efficient ways to become proficient in a trade without needing to take a lot of unnecessary academic courses. Rita completed her tax preparer training through a course offered by the IRS.

The School of Hard Knocks: Life is the best teacher, and sometimes we learn more from our mistakes than we do from success. However, it's easy for young women to neglect to realize how educated they are in life. For example, Kisha thought of herself as uneducated, but when she went to the computer training school, one of her mentors there helped her see that in being a mother she had learned a lot of skills. If she viewed her little family as a business, with income and expenses, she had a lot of management skills. She realized that in her own way she had considerable experience in time and people management and in budgeting.

The final reason to get educated is that it can be fun. If it feels as if your education stopped after you left college, then a self-schooling program might rekindle the fires of learning in your soul. Taking skiing lessons, learning another language, joining a book study group, learning mountain climbing or sailing, taking an acting class, or learning to cook Chinese food can all be fun ways to enrich your life. Being comfortable with learning, and looking at it as an opportunity and a challenge rather than a struggle, will open your eyes to how much learning you have already done and how much more rich your life can be if you continue to learn.

6
Make the Connection: Decide to Be an Effective Communicator

***

Can we talk?

—Joan Rivers

***

No matter how educated, intelligent and capable you are, if you can't communicate what you know, you won't be able to use it effectively. I attended a lecture by a communications consultant who asked her large audience, "How many of you are public speakers?" A few raised their hands. "Oh," she said, "The rest of you speak only to yourselves?" Everyone laughed, but her point was made. We all speak in public every day, and it is every bit as important for you to reach your audience as it is for the highest paid professional lecturer.

Different women have trouble communicating effectively for different reasons:

Rita, because she only completed high school and spent most of her time with her small children, hesitates to offer opinions and join in conversations because she feels uneducated and unsure of herself.

Kim, because her family came from another culture, sometimes worries that what she has to say will sound foreign or strange to her fellow students, professors and friends.

Jodie, because she wound up managing people in her own company at an early age, often feels at a loss about how to talk to her employees who are sometimes older and more experienced.

Kisha, because her lack of education and disadvantaged background have limited her experience, is often intimidated around people who have done and seen more.

Robin, because her dysfunctional family didn't talk about any real issues and argued rather than discussed problems, often feels at a loss about what "normal" people would say in an unfamiliar or tough situation.

Sharon, with her excellent education, worries that her problems finding a good job after she got her MBA mean she isn't communicating effectively.

Because we learn to talk as a gradual process beginning in early infancy, *how* we communicate seems automatic and somewhat mysterious. We speak naturally in the style and manner of the people who surround us, because we learn by imitation. If our parents and family are educated and well-spoken, we'll sound like they do, which can be an advantage, but even educated people may not be good at communicating about personal issues, solving problems or confronting each other effectively when necessary.

Communication is a skill, like many others you have learned, and there are techniques, rules and guidelines you can learn to help you communicate more effectively. By becoming proficient at communication, you will make it easier to achieve your goals when other people are involved.

Almost every woman can benefit from improving her communication skills, in personal relationships as well as business and professional situations. We need to know how to communicate with different people with different styles and in various situations, under pressure and with humor.

Communication skills are valuable in all walks of life. The ability to understand and be understood is the basis for all success, whether in family relationships, business transactions or day-to-day interactions with all kinds of people.

THE BASICS OF COMMUNICATION

Effective communication involves many techniques, including being clear and choosing the right time and place. There are many ways to learn good communication techniques, from joining Toastmasters to taking classes in communication. Search the Internet for referrals to some appropriate organizations.

Although the scope of this book prevents teaching all of the necessary communication skills, I will include the following guidelines for two of the most effective communication techniques, "active listening" and "attentive speaking." These are among the most basic and universal skills and will improve all of your communication.

Active Listening

"Speaking is a dialogue, not a prologue," says communication expert, Alice Weiser, "You can never get into trouble from over-listening."

Active listening is a technique designed to help you *hear* the other person better. When you want to be sure you hear what someone else is saying, and you also want them to *know* that you understand, active listening can help you. Active listening means paying attention to the other person the way you'd like him or her to pay attention to what you say. To do this, you paraphrase (repeat in your own words) what he or she says to demonstrate that you are listening carefully and to verify that you understand what was meant.

Guidelines for Active Listening

Learn to recognize when the discussion is significant. While some people have no problem saying, "I have something important to tell you," most of us usually aren't so clear. Sometimes, the significance of the conversation is obvious from the content, as when you are discussing an important business deal or whether or not to get married. Other times, the clues come from the other person, and you can tell from his or her seriousness or nervousness. Of course, if the other person picks the time and place carefully, or if it is someone important to you, those are also reasons for active listening.

1. **Show you are paying attention to what the other person is saying.** *You know you have succeeded in understanding what the other person means when you can repeat what you heard and the other person agrees. For example, if he or she says, "The contract will be signed on Friday," you can reply, "That's this Friday, here in the office?" When the other person says "yes" or nods, you both know the communication is complete. If you somehow misunderstood, the other person has an opportunity to correct the information.*

2. **Ask questions if you don't understand.** *If your colleague is going on at length, you might say, "Could you stop a minute? I want to be sure I understand your last point before you go on to the next." Then repeat what you have heard so far and get confirmation that you heard it correctly. Don't allow yourself to become overwhelmed by a torrent of words or confusing statements; ask for explanations when you need them.*

3. **Remember that listening carefully does not necessarily mean you agree.** *Even if you find that you disagree, you'll have a better chance of negotiating successfully if you have a clear understanding of the opposing ideas. Saying, "Tell me more," is a wonderful way to be*

attentive when you are not sure you agree but want to understand what is going on before you question or challenge the other person. You may find that you simply misunderstood, or that you're not as opposed as you thought.

4. **Take responsibility for speaking and listening.** *If it seems to you that active listening means you have to take responsibility for both sides of the conversation, you're right, to a degree. Communication works best when both speaker and listener take responsibility for being heard and for hearing. While this may sound like a lot of work in the beginning, it will soon become obvious how much easier it is than not communicating.*

Attentive Speaking

The second component of effective communication is attentive speaking. Although a lot has been written about active listening, attentive speaking is less well-known and less understood. It is a technique taught mostly to salespeople and public speakers to help them keep the attention of their customers or audiences, and to make them more aware of whether they're getting their ideas across (so they can convince more effectively, and thus sell more). It is a simple and highly effective technique that will help you communicate better with everyone you know.

Attentive speaking simply means paying attention, not only to what *you* are saying but also to how the other person is *receiving* it. If you watch carefully when you want to get a point across, the other person's facial expression, body movements and posture will provide clues to help you know whether you are being understood (looking interested, fidgeting, looking bored, eyes wandering, attempting to interrupt, facial expressions of anger or confusion, or a blank, empty stare).

By using the following guidelines, you can learn to observe the listener and determine whether you are successfully communicating without needing any verbal communication from your listener. This is especially effective if the other person is not very talkative, is reluctant to disagree or object, is the strong, silent type, is easily overwhelmed in a discussion, or is passive.

Sometimes listeners are reluctant to let you know they disagree. If you don't use attentive speaking to see the clues, you can be chattering blithely when the listener suddenly reacts with anger, misunderstands you or is just not interested in listening any more—and all your efforts to communicate are wasted. Attentive speaking will help you achieve the following:

- avoid overwhelming the other person with too much information at once (because you will notice when he or she looks overwhelmed, bored or distracted);

- keep your listener's interest in what you have to say (by teaching you how to ask a question when you see his or her attention slipping away);

- understand when what you say is misunderstood (by observing facial expressions and noticing when they're different from what you expect);

- gauge your listener's reaction when he or she doesn't say anything (by facial expressions, body language and attentiveness); and,

- recognize when the other person is too distracted, stressed or preoccupied to really hear what you're saying (by facial expressions, body language and attentiveness).

By using the guidelines that follow, you can figure out when you aren't communicating well or getting the reaction you want.

Guidelines for Attentive Speaking

1. **Watch your listener.** *When it is important to communicate effectively, be careful not to get so engrossed in what you are saying that you forget to watch your listener. Keeping your eyes on your listener's face and body will: (a) let him/her know you care if he or she hears you and (b) increase your listener's tendency to make eye contact and listen more carefully.*

2. **Look for clues in your listener's facial expression** *(a smile, a frown, a glassy-eyed stare), body position (upright and alert, slumped and sullen, turned away from you and inattentive) and movements (leaning toward you, pulling away from you, fidgeting, restless).*

*For example, if you say, "You did a great job,"
and you observe that your listener turns away
and looks out the window, you are getting clues
that you weren't received the way you wanted.
Either the other person is too distracted to hear
you or is having a problem with what you said.*

3. **Ask; don't guess.** *If you get a response that
seems unusual or inappropriate to what you
said (you think you're giving a compliment and
the listener looks confused, hurt or angry; or
you think you're stating objective facts and he or
she appears to be disagreeing; or you're angry
but your listener is smiling), ask a gentle
question—for example, "I thought I was giving
you a compliment, but you look annoyed. Did I
say something wrong?" Or, "Gee, I thought you'd
be happy to hear this but you look upset. Please
tell me what you're thinking." Or, "I'm angry
about what you just said, but you're smiling. Did
I misunderstand you?" Or, "Do you agree?"*

4. **Give your listener a choice.** *If your listener
becomes fidgety or looks off into space as you
talk, either what you're saying is uncomfortable
for your listener, the time is not good for talking
(business pressures, stress, the ball game is on),
the listener is bored or you've been talking too
long. If you think you've been talking too long or
your listener looks bored, invite a comment:
"What do you think?" or, "Do you see it the same
way?" or, "Am I talking too much (or too fast)?"
If you think it's a bad time, ask about it: "You*

look distracted. Is this a good time to talk about this?" (If it is a bad time, then make a date to talk at a better time, or just begin again later.)

5. **Be aware of confusion.** *When you're paying attention as you speak, incomprehension and confusion are easy to spot. If your listener begins to exhibit a blank or glassy-eyed look, or looks worried or confused, you may be putting out too many ideas at once, or you may not be explaining your thoughts clearly. Again, ask a question: "Am I making sense to you?" "Am I going too fast?" "Do you have any questions?" Sometimes, a pause will give the listener the room needed to ask a question and clear up confusion.*

Paying close attention to your listener(s) will make a big difference in the effectiveness of your speaking on a personal or public level. If your listener begins to get lost, bored or confused, you will know it right away and can fix the problem instantly. In addition, after following active listening and attentive speaking guidelines enough to become comfortable with the techniques, you'll find you have greater confidence in your ability to communicate well. This increased faith in your ability will make it much easier for you to meet new people and handle business and personal challenges with confidence.

***Sharon** was well qualified with an MBA, but her job search was not going well, so she took a communication workshop to improve her* *presentation in interviews. "I improved my communication, and now I feel more effective, and much more secure at an interview."*

Rita *gladly took an offer at her work to attend a communication workshop, and improve her adult conversational skills, since her conversations at home were mostly with children. "I feel so much more confident now in conversations with colleagues. I understand better, I'm sure I'm understood, and I offer my own opinion with authority. I even do better with my children."*

Kim *signed up for communications classes because of her worry that she sounded foreign. "I thought I had an accent, but the teacher said I sounded fine. I did learn about cultural communication differences, and I'm more sure of myself. Now I want to practice pediatrics with children of dual cultures, like me."*

Jodie *needs excellent communication skills to manage employees, and settle disputes and customer complaints. She hires a communication expert to teach employee workshops, and got private coaching for herself. "I sponsor workshops in employee teamwork and customer relations, and it's the best money I ever spent. We're a service business, and better communication means better service."*

Kisha *improved her grammar and learned some basic communication techniques with software from the Internet, but wanted more. Her case worker referred her to a class in work-*

related communication skills. "I learned a more formal style of work communication; and I don't feel out of place at work anymore."

Robin knew her dysfunctional family's argumentative style was ineffective, so she worked on a more effective problem solving style in therapy and workshops. "The more I learned about personal communicating and problem-solving, the better I was in other settings— with clients, colleagues, and lecturing. Communication is better everywhere in my life."

Communication skills vary from simply learning to express yourself clearly to complex studies of body language and psychology. Often, a subtle difference in your expression of an idea can make a big difference in how well it is received. Appropriate humor, for example, can ease a tense situation. Becoming a good and skillful communicator, in both talking and listening, gets others enthused about your ideas and decisions.

SOCIAL COMMUNICATION FOR FUN AND STIMULATION

Effective communication skills help you connect with important people. It's a tool for solving problems and achieving goals, but used socially, it is also our most common form of entertainment.

Kisha left high school when she became pregnant. Consequently, she felt intimidated and inadequate in new situations and when meeting new people. Bright as she was, she often felt stupid around more educated people. Once the conversation strayed from work or classes, it would move to all kinds of topics which were a mystery to Kisha. While lively conversation went on all about her, she was silent and uncomfortable.

Once you establish effective communication techniques, you need information to share to be enjoyable and interesting to others. Knowing you can discuss popular topics adds to your confidence and ease in social settings. Whether you are chatting with coworkers, at lunch with clients, relaxing with friends, or even on vacation around total strangers, you can become a source of great conversation. Knowledge of current events, the arts, entertainment, science and technology, politics, or sports provides the material you need to be a social success.

It may surprise you to learn there's fun in the news: it's not all about disasters, politics, world conflicts and depressing events. News is also about art, theater, interesting cultural developments and exciting scientific and medical breakthroughs. There is much power in being informed: besides becoming a great conversationalist, you can keep up with the latest in your fields of interest, be constantly stimulated with new ideas, and able to relate to everyone on many subjects.

THE NATIONAL SALON

Social contact, especially in business settings, is largely based on discussing topics that are part of what is called the "national salon." Salons are social gatherings for the purpose of having stimulating discussions. Interesting events that are publicized in the national media (world affairs, sports, the arts, bestselling books, movies, TV specials, scientific innovations and political or cultural issues) become topics that socially aware people know, and can discuss during business meetings, parties, and other gatherings of people who do not know each other well. Your ability to keep up in such discussions may affect how successful you are at making a good impression on new acquaintances, business associates and clients. Much social and business success has been achieved by women who can keep a lively discussion going.

Becoming well versed in the national salon topics is easier than it may seem. As a reader, probably the most pleasant way for you to become informed and up-to-date is to subscribe to a national news magazine, some of which are free online. Just do a search for "National News Magazines." If you don't like news of war, politics or international events, try reading the last half of the magazine, which is devoted to news about the arts and sciences, medical and science breakthroughs, technical innovations, interesting people and book and movie reviews.

***Kisha** confided her frustration to a friend from computer training, who suggested either subscribing to a national magazine or reading one regularly at the library. The magazine was expensive for Kisha, so she borrowed a copy from a friend. "Even reading that one issue opened my eyes," says Kisha. "What people were talking about was explained in detail in the magazine."*

She began to read magazines in the library, and she read articles online during her work breaks.

After a while, Kisha felt brave enough to join the conversations her coworkers were having. She no longer felt isolated once she began talking and having fun with her office mates.

Being a good communicator involves continuous learning. In the next chapter, we'll see how important lifelong learning is, and how much fun it can be.

7
Be Young in Mind:
Decide to Keep Learning

It's never too late to be what you might have been.

—George Eliot

Getting an education is important for most of us. As we discussed in chapter 5, there are many kinds of education, formal and informal, that can be useful in following your road map and reaching your chosen destination. Even after you meet your initial education and training goals, you'll still find that learning has benefits. Lifelong learning involves keeping yourself informed about the health, financial and political issues that affect you, your career, your finances, your future and your family. Being informed gives you an advantage in every aspect of your life. On the job, in social settings, with your family and your children, and for your own pleasure, learning is one way to keep yourself young and vital, throughout your entire life. If you're interested in many things, you will be more interesting to those around you, and even to yourself.

Current research in the psychology of happiness and optimal experience, as conducted by Dr. Mihaly Csikszentmihalyi of the University of Chicago, indicates that people who are doing new tasks are happier and more fulfilled. "People who [have] the drive to be independent and autonomous... are fully individualized, unique, interesting," he writes in *The Evolving Self*. ". . . 'Flow' [the kinds of experiences that focus our whole being in a harmonious rush of energy, and lift us out of the anxieties and boredom that characterize so much of everyday life] usually happens... when we are actively involved in a difficult enterprise, in a task that stretches our physical and mental abilities."

According to Harvard researcher Dr. Ellen Langer, an active, learning mind enhances health and even reverses some of the effects formerly attributed to aging: "...the receiving of new information is a basic function of living creatures. In fact, lack of new information can be harmful... the sensory system often shuts down, since it is not 'receiving' anything new," warns Dr. Langer, in her book *Mindfulness*. "Success in increasing longevity by making more cognitive demands... or by teaching meditation or techniques of flexible, novel thinking gives us strong reason to believe that the same techniques could be used to improve health and shorten illness earlier in life.... The research... shows that mindfulness leads to feelings of control, greater freedom of action, and less burnout."

BECOME YOUR OWN ENCYCLOPEDIA

Your brain is a remarkable resource: it sorts, stores and retrieves all kinds of information.

Marie has memorized a lot of music: popular songs, folk tunes, religious and classical arias. Now that she has stored all of this music in her mind, she finds that she can retrieve it in many ways: if she hears a piece on the radio, she can recognize it and remember the title, the composer and the work it is from; if she thinks of a tempo, such as waltz time, she can remember most of the pieces she knows that are waltzes; she can also remember pieces in other categories, such as by composer, by language, by subject matter or other characteristics, such as all the arias in a particular opera; and she also can recall specifics such as when she learned a song or a whole repertoire for a particular concert or recital.

Marie has done the work of memorizing all this musical information, but once that work is done her brain organizes and retrieves it automatically, and your brain helps you in the same way.

If you learn to use it well, this personal encyclopedia can help you in a lot of ways: You can store and retrieve technical information you use in your career, such as computer programming languages or accounting procedures; you can recall entertaining jokes, stories and anecdotes on the spot to liven up a conversation or perk up a boring business meeting; you can store and use information about current events, historical facts, interesting commentary heard on the radio or fascinating facts gleaned from the Internet to make your general conversation more stimulating and enjoyable; and you can store and retrieve observations of your daily life and the habits and quirks of others to create a novel, a work of art, a comedy routine, a screenplay or a memoir.

You can use the marvelous capacity of your mind to store information for work and for play. You must choose information you wish to store in your personal encyclopedia, because you will never run out of room.

While it takes work to memorize a lot of information, being interested and informed can do some of the job for you. If you choose some areas of special interest (such as national salon topics, parenting information, technical information useful in your profession or information pertaining to hobbies) and regularly read in those subject areas, you'll find that your interest alone is enough to help you retain the information. Also, reading regularly in a field means you will encounter certain basic facts over and over, and the repetition will help you retain the information.

General information can be enough for you to know in order to participate in an interesting discussion of the economy with colleagues in your line of business; it is probably enough to know some information about trends and events. If, on the other hand, you are making important business decisions or giving a presentation or seminar, you need more details and hard facts.

There are many resources for facts and information that are surprisingly easy to access.

USE THE LIBRARY AND THE INTERNET

If you have access to the Internet, there may be a way for you to customize your starting page in a way that accesses online news media and alerts you to the stories of the day in the topics you select (sports, fashion, the arts, finance, world affairs, etc.). On the Internet, you may also search for any topic that interests you. By clicking on the "search" button on your Internet browser and following the instructions, or accessing a search engine of your choice, you can research any subject. You can also locate people or businesses by using online search engines. You'll find an overwhelming amount of information very easily, so narrow your search.

If you can't access the Internet at home, school or work, try to access it at your public library, which also is still the best repository of books and information around. Don't hesitate to ask the librarian for information or assistance. In your local library, you can find the equivalent of a complete education on almost any subject, and your library staff can network with others to obtain books that your local branch doesn't have, or help you with your search.

If reading is difficult for you because of poor eyesight, dyslexia or another problem, many books and magazines are available on tape or on computers and other devices that can read written text to you. Libraries are excellent sources for CD-ROMs, CDs, audio- and videotapes, and books on tape.

In addition to your local public library, if there is a college or university nearby it will also have an excellent library, especially in relationship to subjects that are taught there. If you are not a student, you still may be allowed to use the library, and at some colleges and universities nonstudents, especially if they are local residents, can obtain a library card and check-out privileges for a nominal fee. College libraries usually keep copies of published research and are good places to search for the most recent research in a particular field.

Independent research and study will help you learn and can help you stay healthy, too. In the library, in your local bookstore, in specialized newsletters and magazines, and on the Internet you can find information about the best ways to maintain optimum health. While independent research is not a good substitute for a doctor's advice, it can be an excellent supplement to what a doctor says. Often people who have health problems, from allergies to serious illnesses, find that searching the Internet or the library gives them lots of information they were not able to get from their doctors.

You can explore alternative healing methods, such as shiatsu, acupuncture, acupressure, chiropractic, herbal medicine, homeopathy and the other alternative therapies. Your research can provide answers to your questions about which modalities are right for you, whether you want to maintain your health or resolve a health problem.

Rita's little girl, Susie, has skin rashes, upper respiratory infection, and allergies to certain foods and other irritants. When Rita was dissatisfied with the advice she got from Susie's pediatrician, she found an Internet "chat-room" discussion on children's illnesses and discovered remedies and dietary changes that greatly helped Susie. "I didn't use all the advice I was given," says Rita, "I checked with Susie's doctor, and cautiously began to follow some of the suggestions. Some worked for Susie, some didn't— but I was able to try things I never would have known about if I had not found the online forum. Also, when I was worried, it was wonderful to have so much support."

READING FOR MENTAL AND PHYSICAL WELL-BEING

Using books to fix your relationship, personal, health and emotional problems has become such a common thing for people to do today that it even has a name: bibliotherapy. There are huge numbers of fine-quality psychology/self-help and health-related books available everywhere today. It is relatively easy to become your own expert by reading the research and advice of experts you probably couldn't otherwise access.

While books alone won't be sufficient to help you solve severe emotional, stress or relationship problems, they can certainly help you with lesser problems. Reading books relating to your issues can enhance the therapy process, helping you to understand the problems and the solutions better, and thereby saving you time and money in therapy. You can also feel supported by knowing others have faced similar problems.

__Megan__ wanted to reduce her stress, and went to the library to do some research. After reading a few books on stress reduction, she decided to try *yoga. She wanted to practice at home, and didn't have enough time for classes. At the library, she found yoga books and videotapes for beginners; she tried several until she found one she could follow easily. There were also YouTube instruction videos. When she found a video series she liked online, she was able to practice regularly on her own, for a year. "At the end of that year," she says, "I wanted to make yoga a permanent part of my life, because it really helped reduce my stress, and my body was feeling much better; and I read that it could keep me supple and healthy into my old age, which sounded like a great idea. So, I searched again until I found a teacher I liked, at a time I could attend."*

Whether you are looking for the proper way to develop a new relationship, solve communication problems, reduce emotional stress, or understand your grief, anger, anxiety or depression, books are likely to have the answers you seek. If you are discouraged, anxious or lonely, a book can offer reassurance, support and comfort when friends and family are unavailable. There are many motivational and inspirational books that can give you a boost, lift your spirits and encourage you when you are struggling.

Books also are a great resource for keeping up with the national salon.

***Jodie**'s business success happened so quickly that she never went to college, and consequently felt left out of discussions about classic literature and* *history. So she decided to read at night. Online, she found a list of the "Great Books of the Western World" and read many, then asked her librarian for recommendations. Soon the librarian had books set aside for Jodie when she came in. Jodie began to watch the bestsellers lists and book reviews herself, and read whatever interested her. "I learned a lot about history, culture and psychology, and soon was a star in those discussions that used to intimidate me. Now, I love reading and I can join a discussion on any subject."*

YOUR LEARNING STYLE

Reading is not the only way to learn. Different people learn in different ways. Just as you have your own style of living and your preferred way of dress, you also have certain ways of absorbing information. There are four ways we acquire information—*auditory* (hearing), *visual* (seeing), *tactile* (touching) and *imaginative* (thinking). Most of us learn by using a combination of these avenues, and your particular combination becomes your learning style.

Learning is much easier if you know your learning style. If you know how you learn, you can design your lifelong education in whatever way makes it easier. After doing the following exercises, you will have more understanding of how you learn and how to design a program for yourself that makes lifelong learning easy and fun for you.

Each new thing you learn changes your perception of yourself and your environment: it is exciting to see things from a new perspective. Realizing how rewarding learning is increases your motivation to learn, and through learning, you obtain new options and solutions to old problems, which will make your decisions easier.

Many people think of learning as work, but most of our learning takes place without our even being aware of it. For example, as a newborn baby, you had instincts, emotions and reactions, but you had not yet acquired any habits, attitudes or beliefs. Everything you know today, including speech, and walking, you learned without knowing you were learning. It's only when we are taught that learning is hard work, as in school, that we resist it. In order to pursue lifelong learning easily, as Jon Spayde writes in his article "The New Renaissance" we must go back to the old viewpoint:

"Suppose we abandon the notion that learning is time-consuming and obligatory, and replaced it with the idea, courtesy of Goethe, that 'people cannot learn what they do not love'—the idea of learning as an encounter infused with Eros. We always find time for what we truly love, one way or another. Suppose further, that love, being an inclusive spirit, refused to choose between Shakespeare and Toni Morrison (or Tony Bennet, for that matter), and we located our bliss in the unstable relationship between the two, rattling from book to book, looking for connections and grandly unconcerned about whether we've read enough as long as we read what we read with love... The whole world's a classroom, and to really make it one, the first thing is to believe it is."

You continually learn new things, whether it's learning a new job or playing a sport. And, you have learned these things in your own unique way: slightly different from the way someone else would do it. Therefore, the question is not to teach you how to learn, but to help you discover how you naturally learn: your personal learning style.

LEARNING HOW YOU LEARN

Learning becomes easier and more effective when you become aware of how you learn. People receive information in different ways: we are auditory, visual, tactile and imaginative in different proportions. That is, words (sounds), pictures (sight), touch and imagination are more or less important to each of us depending upon our learning styles. Your learning style consists of two parts: sensory preference and attitude. Sensory preference is merely a description of which senses you naturally use more than others. Learning attitude is a more complex description of how your personality traits, learning history and prejudices affect your approach to learning. Together, they comprise your learning style.

Sensory Preference

Sensory preference refers to the senses that help you learn most easily and with the deepest understanding, such as the following:

- *Auditory:* If you absorb information mostly through listening to words and you think in words rather than pictures, your style is more verbal and auditory and not very visual. In visualization exercises, you will be more likely to think in words than in pictures, and you know you have learned a new idea when you can explain it clearly. It would be most effective for you to talk, hear or read about new ideas, and lectures and audiotapes may be a good way for you to learn. You may enjoy listening to the radio. You'll probably use a phrase like: "I hear what you're saying," or "It sounds like..." to mean you understand someone.

- *Visual:* If you understand better when you see things, and you tend to picture ideas rather than think them in words, you probably know you've learned something only when you can visualize the steps or imagine yourself using them effectively. Visualization techniques, videos, watching someone else, or using diagrams and pictures are probably the most effective way for you to learn. You may say visual things like "I see," meaning, "I understand," or "See that?" meaning, "Do you understand?"

- *Tactile:* If you lean toward the physical and you are a tactile (touching) person, you learn best by doing, by tinkering with things, and you know you've learned it when you feel it more than see or hear it. "Walking through" a new skill or habit, acting it out physically, works well for you. For you, "I feel it," or "I've got it," are ways to say you understand.

- *Imaginative:* Are you a daydreamer? Do you often practice scenes in your imagination such as playing over a job interview in your head before you actually go on one? For you, "I wonder," "Let me think about it," and "I can see it in my mind's eye," are common statements.

No matter what learning style suits you best, if you take advantage of your sensory preference learning will be easier for you because you will not have to struggle against or translate the method you're learning from into your own preference before you can absorb the information.

Learning Attitude

Attitude is the other part of your learning style. Your attitude is heavily influenced by your early environment and experience and refers to the pre-set ideas you have before you encounter new information. Some people are enthusiastic about learning because their experiences in the past were rewarding; some people are more cautious; and some people are resistant because learning meant failure in the past (like a bad school experience). Your learning attitude also includes preferences (whether you like to learn quickly or slowly, alone or with others) and prejudices, such as, "Book learning is more prestigious than learning a trade."

These attitude differences can be incorporated in your learning in the same way you use your sensory preferences.

For example, if you like to learn with others and you think "book learning" is best, you can form a book study group. If you like to learn alone and you value practical learning (skills you use), you'll enjoy video- or audiotapes or books with titles that begin with "How to..." or an Internet search.

Some learning attitudes can create problems. If you come from a family where education is emphasized positively, your attitude toward organized learning will be positive. You'll be proud of formal, organized learning (schools, courses), anticipate it with excitement and seek it out. However, your family may value academics above sports, current events, mechanics and the arts, which may cause you to miss the fact that there are many kinds of learning.

If you come from a family where education is laughed at, or where you're told you're stupid, or if you were pressured too hard to learn in school, book learning will have been emphasized negatively and you'll fear it. However, you may be much better and more relaxed at other activities, such as auto mechanics or dance—they are kinds of learning, too.

Your attitude determines whether you approach learning new things with enthusiasm, procrastination, calm or anxiety. Positive attitudes toward particular kinds of learning make those easier to process ("I love school, and it's fun and easy." "I love to work with my hands."), and negative attitudes make particular kinds more difficult ("I hate getting my hands dirty." "I'm afraid of hurting myself." "I'm not good at anything mechanical." "I hate books and teachers." "I was never good at school.").

If your family created pressure about school grades or caused you to feel that learning was for "sissies," you may try to avoid it. (It's impossible to avoid learning, but if you have a rigid definition of what learning is, you can believe you do avoid it.) If you attempt to avoid learning, you may wind up learning many new things "the hard way," through being forced to by negative experiences. That is, if you don't learn about your car because it's "dirty work" you may be cheated by mechanics, left stranded on the highway, etc., until you learn enough to know the danger signs of a failing car.

The following quizzes are intended to help you discover your learning style: the first one is about sensory preference and the second is about learning attitude. After taking them, you'll combine them both to form a complete learning profile, which you can then use to make all future learning easier. There are no right or wrong answers. You may have more than one choice per question, or a more appropriate, original answer. No one is 100 percent auditory, visual, tactile or imaginative. We experience with all four of these senses, but we have preferences.

Quiz 1: Sensory Preference

Take a sheet of paper and make four headings across the top. Down the left-hand margin, write the numbers 1 to 5, as shown below:

Auditory   Visual   Tactile   Imaginative

1. _____

2. _____

3. _____

4. _____

5. _____

Make a check mark in the category you choose for each answer to the following questions. When you're done, tally your totals. The category with the most check marks will indicate the sensory mode through which you learn most easily. The columns with the highest number of check marks indicate your natural learning modes (the senses through which you learn readily), and those with the fewest check marks indicate modes that are less easy for you to use. The results indicate what your most natural, habitual and effective sensory preferences are. Tailor your own learning experiences to take advantage of your style.

1. When you think, you:
    (a) hear words in your head (auditory).
    (b) draw or visualize pictures (visual).
    (c) write things down or touch related objects (tactile).
    (d) daydream fantasies and visions (imaginative).
2. When you are or were in school, you learned better from teachers who:
    (a) gave interesting talks and told stories (auditory).
    (b) wrote or drew diagrams on the board or showed movies and pictures (visual).
    (c) gave you hands-on experiments or homework (tactile).
    (d) asked you to imagine or guess what the situation was like (imaginative).
3. When you want to learn something new (for example, operating a computer, cooking Chinese food, a new game or sport) you:

(a) take a class or read a book *(auditory)*.

(b) watch someone else do it first *(visual)*.

(c) experiment and learn as you go *(tactile)*.

(d) dream about knowing how to do it *(imaginative)*.

4. You feel confident you've learned something when you:

(a) can explain it to someone *(auditory)*.

(b) can see the results or watch yourself do well in a mirror or video *(visual)*.

(c) do it with your own hands, or when it "feels" easy *(tactile)*.

(d) can see yourself doing it well in your imagination *(imaginative)*.

5. You do a lot of:

(a) reading and writing *(auditory)*.

(b) watching TV, movies, people *(visual)*.

(c) physical activity *(tactile)*.

(d) daydreaming, fantasizing *(imaginative)*.

After marking your answers and tallying them, take the next quiz, in which you will use your sensory preference from Quiz 1.

Quiz 2: Learning Attitude

Your learning attitude is more ambiguous than your sensory preference and does not lend itself to columns of check marks, as did Quiz 1. Heading a piece of paper "How I Learn" and writing your answers out will give you a more useful, narrative description of your style. For example, if your answer to question 1 below is (a), write it out as "I approach learning something new with *an 'Oh, boy' attitude." When you've written out all the answers, you'll have a paragraph that describes your learning attitude. You will find a sample paragraph and instructions for how to use it at the end of the quiz.*

1. *You approach learning with an:*
   (a) *"Oh, boy!" attitude.*
   (b) *"Oh, dear" attitude.*
   (c) *"So what" attitude.*
2. *While reading this book, you feel:*
   (a) *skepticism.*
   (b) *acceptance.*
   (c) *resistance.*
   (d) *desperation.*
3. *When you first encountered this exercise, you:*
   (a) *read the whole thing through without doing it (to know what it was about before you did it).*
   (b) *pluged right in and did it as you went along.*
   (c)*shared it with a friend first to see his or her reaction.*
4. *You feel learning is:*
   (a) *work.*
   (b) *helpful.*
   (c) *fun.*
   (d) *like solving a puzzle.*
5. *You often:*
   (a) *get lost in learning something new and forget what time it is.*
   (b) *learn something new just to make life more fun and interesting.*
   (c) *have to have a logical reason to learn something.*
   (d) *resist or procrastinate about learning.*

6. When learning new things, you are most motivated to:
   (a) prove you can do it.
   (b) compete with someone.
   (c) beat your own previous effort.
   (d) make a good impression.

7. When you face a brand-new task, you prefer:
   (a) to be left alone until you figure it out.
   (b) to be led, step-by-step through it until you know it.
   (c) a combination of guidance and hands-on practice.
   (d) to have written instructions.

8. What seems more valuable to you?
   (a) things people learn from books, teachers and/or school.
   (b) "trades" people learn, such as mechanics or carpentry.
   (c) what people learn in office jobs.
   (d) practical skills like driving or cooking.
   (e) fun skills like sports, the arts or hobbies.

9. Rank the answers from question 8 in order of their value or importance to you as follows:
   (a) most important (write in a, b, c, d or e from question 8).
   (b) very important.
   (c) somewhat important.
   (d) not very important.
   (e) least important.

10. Now rank the same answers from question 8 in order of their usefulness to you:
    (a) most useful (a, b, c, d or e from question 8).

(b) very useful.

(c) somewhat useful.

(d) not very useful.

(e) least useful.

11. *I know I have learned enough (for now) when I:*

(a) feel overwhelmed and confused by new information.

(b) have mastered the new task or skill.

(c) am told it's time to take a break.

(d) get bored and restless.

(e) feel _____(fill in the blank).

At the end of your paragraph, add the information from the first quiz. Remember: Preference + Attitude = Learning Style. Following is an example of Kim's result from the two quizzes.

How **Kim** learns:

I approach learning with an "Oh, dear" attitude. Even while reading this book I feel resistance. When I first encountered this exercise, I read the whole thing through without doing it because I was nervous about it. I feel learning is helpful, but I often resist or procrastinate about learning. When learning new things, I am most motivated to beat my own previous effort. When I face a brand-new task, I prefer to be led, step-by-step through it until I know it. The most valuable learning to me is what people learn from teachers and school. The most important learning is what people learn in school. The least important learning is the "trades." The most useful learning is what people learn in office jobs, and practical skills like cooking and driving. The least useful are the "trades." I know I have learned enough when I feel overwhelmed and confused by new information. My learning style is mostly visual, somewhat imaginative and not auditory at all.

Now complete your paragraph. When you are done, read the paragraph out loud onto tape. Using your individual sensory preference, either: listen to it or discuss it with a friend (auditory); act it out in front of a mirror (visual); make a mental picture of yourself learning in different ways (imaginative); or put the components of your style on index cards you can reorganize in several different ways, or, if possible, use small items to physically represent the components of your learning style (tactile).

Spend some time thinking about what your learning style means, and the easiest learning experiences you have had. Did they fit your learning style? When you had difficulty learning something, was the method you were using inappropriate to your learning style? For example, auditory learners often find they can't learn in a noisy environment. These people need a quiet environment for studying, and they like to attend lectures and conferences. Visual people like pictures, graphs, watching someone work or learning from videos. Being in a beautiful environment is often important to learning. A teacher with bad taste in clothes can distract them from what they are learning. Imaginative people don't like to be rushed, or to be required to have an instant answer. They like to mull over the information, imagine themselves using it in different ways and "live" with it for a while. They often love to read descriptive passages in books, poetry, etc. Their mental pictures are so vivid; they can learn from stories. Tactile people don't bother to read directions. They like to get their hands on the information, and—if they are learning something abstract—models they can manipulate or even flash cards they can hold.

After reviewing her paragraph and picturing in her imagination how her learning style would look in action, Kim realized she was very tentative about learning, would do best with a guide or teacher, and most respected institutional (school) learning, although she used practical learning more. "After thinking about my preferences for a while," says Kim, "I decided that using a support group or learning with a friend or taking classes would be easiest for me because I could take the time to visualize the subject I'm learning, or watch someone else, or use pictures such as videos or an illustrated anatomy book, to make learning easier." She also decided to encourage herself more about being able to learn during her daily review.

Like Kim, you can visualize your learning style more clearly and reinforce and support the aspects where you need help. By understanding how you learn and using it to your advantage, you can become more aware of and comfortable with your sensory preferences and learning attitudes, and you can use your learning style to make learning easier and more fun.

Becoming comfortable with and understanding your style of learning can renew and recharge all your decisions. By being self-aware, you can make the most of your style, your assets and liabilities, and your strengths and weaknesses.

As we discovered earlier, good decisions require information and research. If you keep yourself interested and informed, you will already have the facts you need when you want to make any decision, from business to personal. It is not necessary to wait until you have a specific decision to research. The best decision-makers have a fund of knowledge they can draw on instantly, when the need for a quick, effective decision arises. It is through lifelong learning, a love of reading and gaining knowledge that they build the internal resources they can draw on in time of need.

Now that you have a clear picture of your destination, and an understanding of your learning style and what makes good communication and conversation, you are ready to connect with the people around you who can help you reach your goals—and to have fun along the way. The next chapter is about finding and making connections with the people you need to help you get where you want to go.

8
It Takes a Village:
Decide to Build Personal and
Professional Networks

*The healthy and strong individual is
the one who asks for help when she
needs it— whether she's got an abscess
on her knee or her soul.*

—Rona Barrett

Hillary Rodham Clinton's book *It Takes a Village* is probably the most well-known expression of the African proverb, "It takes a village to raise a child." The currently widespread use of the phrase reflects a realization that, because we are such a mobile and fast-paced society, we need to create a sense of community and connectedness, not only to raise children but to function more effectively in all phases of life. Not only does it take a community to raise a child, but living an effective, enjoyable life as an adult also requires support and connections. "We are creatures of community," writes Dr. Dean Ornish in *Love and Survival: The Scientific Basis for the Healing Power of Intimacy.* "Those individuals, societies, and cultures who learned to take care of each other, to love each other, and to nurture relationships with each other during the past several hundred thousand years were more likely to survive than those who did not.... In short, anything that promotes a sense of isolation often leads to illness and suffering. Anything that promotes a sense of love and intimacy, connection and community is healing."

By learning to find and use the community resources around you, you will set up a network of information and resources that will help you more successfully follow your roadmap and reach your chosen destination.

SUPPORT AND BACKUP

We have all heard that "it's not what you know, it's who you know." To a large extent it's true. Having a widespread network can assist you in many ways. Once established, your network can give you a social support group that's big enough to meet all your social needs; serve as a resource for business, educational and personal connections that will enhance your life in all these areas; provide a number of role models, mentors and teachers; and surround you with a peer group who will understand and support what you are trying to accomplish.

There is no better support network than a large, loving family. Unfortunately, your family may be too small, too far away or too difficult. If you don't have a large extended family, or if your family has no experience in your career area, or if there are not enough family members who are compatible with you, then creating a support network is a must.

> ***Robin*** *was estranged from her family because of their alcoholism and dysfunction. She saw them rarely and could not count on them for support. She felt alone and insecure. She had recurring dreams that something would go wrong, and she'd wind up on the streets as a bag lady. She decided she needed a support network. Through her schooling, and in Al-Anon, she met many friends. As she began to train as an alcoholism counselor, her friends introduced her to other counselors and helped her with her studies. She joined a local branch of the Alcoholism Counselors of America, and at its meetings she met many colleagues. It was through these colleagues that she got recommendations of schools to attend and also found a placement as an intern. Her friends and colleagues provided the support and encouragement she couldn't get from her family. "Once my network was established and strong," Robin says, "I knew that even if I did lose my job and run out of money, I'd be okay. Someone would take me in." Her bad dreams stopped, and she was more able to relax.*

Fortunately, even if you move to a new place for career reasons, you needn't create your network from scratch. Many excellent support networks are pre-established for you, once you learn how to find them and how to use them.

Community and Connectedness

Whether you are in a large or a small community, and whether you grew up in the area or you just moved in, networks that can be helpful to you already exist in your area. Deciding to utilize these connections will enhance both your career and personal life. Most communities have a huge number and variety of social and professional organizations that provide wonderful opportunities to do well by doing good.

By connecting with others, you will gain an enormous pool of resources that make life easier and more pleasant. People working together can make life a lot easier for each other.

Single mothers can share child care, women new in their careers can support each other in learning new tasks, established residents can help newcomers get acquainted and younger people can assist the elderly.

Learning to network makes it possible to create support systems almost instantly in any community, whether you move to a new locale, or travel on business, or just want to have fun in several places. The networks that are already in place can provide instant resources for you, and national networks can give you support networks in places you've never been before.

Social, Service and Religious Organizations

In every community, there are classic organizations, such as: churches and synagogues; Twelve-Step programs; the PTA; Boy Scouts and Girl Scouts; the YWCA; Kiwanis, Rotary and Elks clubs; and the American Association of University Women. Any of these groups can provide a social network if you need one (especially if you're new in town or looking to contact a wider variety of people). Groups in this category exist to fill social and community service and religious functions, but you can use them to provide a ready-made group from which you can make professional, business or social contacts.

> **Sharon** had trouble finding a good job close to home after she got her MBA, so she solved her problem by becoming active in church, and joining the junior chamber of commerce, which helped her get to know the business owners and other important members of her town. Knowing these people, she could find out about new career positions opening and get a personal referral and an interview. Her qualifications and skill at interviewing got her a career-track job she liked, near home. "I found out that in my small city, who I knew was at least as important as my education in finding a job. Once I became active and visible in my church, people offered to help. And, there was the bonus of all the spiritual support."

Becoming involved in social, service and religious groups can give you:

- an opportunity to help others and to influence your community
- emotional and social support for you and your family

- connections with the people who form the "backbone of the community"
- referrals to reliable medical doctors, dentists, auto mechanics, plumbers, real estate or insurance agents, and other useful resources
- inexpensive and available entertainment and social events, with people you know
- an excellent resource for making friends (or even finding a significant relationship) who are known to the others in the group and
- spiritual support and a framework for living a life that is particularly meaningful to you.

When Rita was concerned about whether going back to work was bad for her children, she found a lot of support from other parents in her church. They supported her decision to work part-time and gave her lots of suggestions and ideas for getting organized and making the most of her time with the children.

"Never doubt that a small group of thoughtful, committed citizens can change the world. Indeed it is the only thing that ever has," wrote Margaret Mead in the memoir *With a Daughter's Eye*. While you may or may not be interested in changing the entire world, getting connected with these networks can indeed change your own world for the better.

PROFESSIONAL RESOURCES

Whatever your career, there are professional organizations, such as unions, bar associations, business networking groups like the Chamber of Commerce, and societies like the American Medical Association or the

American Association of Marriage and Family Therapy. Robin used these organizations to make the kinds of connections she needed to support herself in beginning her counseling business.

Professionally focused groups like these: (1) offer education in a specific field (through speakers at meetings, workshops and courses); (2) can connect you with people who are more experienced and who will mentor you; and (3) offer a place for you to ask career-related questions of experts in your field.

Regular attendance at meetings of these organizations will provide you with: up-to-the-minute information about legal changes that affect your career or business; information about new jobs, products, developments or markets; opportunities to hear speakers and attend programs relating directly to your field; and personal connections with the most respected members of your field.

All such groups are listed in your local phone book, at the library or on the Internet. It only takes a phone call to find out the requirements for membership and when the meetings occur. Ask if you can attend as a guest for a while to find out if the group is a good place for you.

National Networks

National professional and social networks offer the added benefit of mobility. The American Society of Journalists and Authors is an unparalleled resource for a nonfiction writer like me. No matter where I plan to go in the United States, I can find members there who recommend the best places to stay, the wonderful little restaurants that only residents know, people to talk to, the best bookstores, and so on. Wherever I am, I can connect with a local chapter for a lively discussion with colleagues who have similar career issues. That's a great resource to have when you're alone and away from home.

National networks can be social or educational, like Mensa or the American Association of University Women; political, like the League of Women Voters or the National Organization for Women; religious, like various church denominations; or career- or business-oriented, like the American Bar Association or the American Society of Women Accountants. Sororities and fraternities have chapters all across the nation, as do all the Twelve-Step groups, such as Alcoholics Anonymous and Co-Dependents Anonymous.

If you're planning to move, or if your firm is relocating you, these national organizations can be priceless. If, for example, you have served on the national board, you'll already be known to members in your new location. Even if you know no one, you can call the local chapter and ask them for recommendations for doctors, real estate agents and other resources.

When Sharon considered moving, she contacted several organizations, from the Methodist Church to the National Association of MBAs to the local Kiwanis and Rotary clubs and the Chamber of Commerce in each city of interest to her. By establishing a phone relationship with members of these organizations, she was able to find out about the climate, the local economy, the opportunities for women and much more before she spent any time in that city. When she decided to visit, she already knew enough that she could choose her hotel and organize her activities for the visit.

A Spiritual Community

We need to be connected, and we often find our connections among friends and family, to whom we feel close because of our similarities, shared history and emotional bonds. In chapter 3, "Where Are You Going?" you had a chance to look at your values and what gives your life meaning. Many successful women build their lives around a core spiritual belief, which may be based on the precepts of an organized religion, such as Protestantism, Judaism, Catholicism, Buddhism or Islam. It also might be based on other kinds of spiritual study, such as a Twelve-Step program, an Oriental art like t'ai chi, a meditative discipline such as transcendental meditation, Sufism or yoga, or a philosophy such as Wicca or Taoism.

If faith is important in your life, then being connected to other members of a church, synagogue, temple or other spiritual group with similar aims and beliefs can support you in living those values. In addition, you can make friends and meet business colleagues in your spiritual community and share friendship and business opportunities with people who have adopted a similar code of ethics and compatible values.

College or University Resources

At a college or a university, the campus will be home to established groups that can be excellent resources. College fraternities, special-interest groups (like computer or language clubs), the school newspaper, honors organizations, and campus political or human-rights organizations are all resources for gathering information and meeting interesting people. Robin and Kisha both used the resources of their respective schools to find support.

School or campus groups allow you to: meet suitable friends who have equal education and similar interests; make friends who might later have influential and powerful careers; learn more than the information presented in your classes (to give yourself an edge over the competition); and get hands-on experience in your chosen career.

To find appropriate campus organizations, read the college catalogue, look in the library and the student affairs office and ask fellow students.

NETWORKING OPTIONS

"As creative children," writes Julia Cameron in *The Artist's Way*, "we are each of us not only instruments but also a note, even a song. When we open our hearts and sing to and with one another, we quite literally create harmony." Learning to create your own network, in addition to the ready-made ones, will bring harmony into your life. There are many kinds of networks you can build.

- *The mommy network*, allows mothers of similar-age children to work together to share carpooling, baby- sitting, information and support. A mommy network made a big difference in **Rita**'s life and career decisions. She got support for her decision to go back to work. The other working mothers helped her find daycare and took turns taking the children overnight so the mom who got the evening off could get some things done, relax or have a quiet evening with her husband. "It was so good for me to know other women who had similar concerns and problems. So many times, when something went wrong, one of the other mothers gave me the help I needed. I don't know what I'd have done without them," remembers Rita.

- *The friends network* provides support and friendship. Getting together with friends you can count on, and meeting new friends or introducing your friends to each other, can build a group with whom you can share holidays, good times, bad times and information. A solid network of friends provides a cushion and a shield in life's difficult times and someone to talk to when you need support or advice. The same network will also make the good times better by celebrating with you and congratulating you. Nothing feels as good in life as being surrounded by a trusted and trustworthy group of friends. Kim's friends helped her evaluate whether medical school was right for her and Megan's friends helped her decide between the mommy track and the career track.

- *The neighbor network* can provide security and enhance your living environment. Knowing your neighbors is becoming increasingly rare, but more and more necessary. Friendly neighbors who know you and your routine are an automatic protection against vandalism and other problems, such as fires and theft, and can even help with package deliveries. In an emergency, a good neighbor will call 911 for you, watch your children or feed your pets. They are much more likely to know if someone is hanging around who doesn't belong in the area. Making friendly gestures toward the people next door, saying "Hi," inviting them for coffee and getting to know them will make your neighborhood a safer and more pleasant place. Your local city councilperson's office or the police can give you the information you need to join or begin a neighborhood watch group. Neighbors include the other residents in your apartment building or condo complex, the people on your block and the ones across the street. Get to know as many as you can.

When **Kisha** had to live in low-income subsidized housing that was not very safe, she and her neighbors organized a neighborhood watch, which helped eliminate drug dealers in the neighborhood. Those same neighbors shared potluck dinners with Kisha and her children and watched her children when she was at school.

- *The family network* can provide all the benefits of friends and neighbors, plus the warmth of a lifetime of love. Not all families qualify as networks. Some siblings and relatives don't get along or support each other. When family functions well, it's great to have people who care about you and really know you. Family is the network we turn to first in times of sickness and financial crisis. If you would like to turn to your family (or some of them) in the tough times, share the good times with them, too. If you appreciate your family, let them know. If you want a good relationship with them, be willing to let them know what kind of contact and support you want. You may be surprised by their response.

If you have problems with certain members of your family, or if they live too far away, try building a partial family network with those family members you like or those who live close. Once you get a small network working smoothly, other family members can be drawn into it. Even though **Kim** feels pressured by her family at times, she loves them and enjoys sharing holidays and achievements and struggles with them.

- *The career and power network* can provide support on the job or getting a job. Friends or college buddies who are well placed can let you know when new jobs arise; coworkers you enjoy can make your day much more pleasant and help you when you need job-related information or support. By utilizing the business networks described earlier, like the chamber of commerce, you can meet people individually and slowly make deeper connections until you have your own career and power business network, made up of people chosen by you for specific reasons.

Robin made excellent use of a professional network to find out about the business side of counseling.

- *The political network* can help you get things done in your community. As with the business network, the quickest way to begin is to get involved in local organizations and pick the individuals you wish to know. Your local city councilor's office has many useful functions, and you can get to know individuals there who can be helpful later. To get connected, work on a campaign (for example, to support a proposition both you and the mayor favor)—you'll meet a lot of the important people in your town or city.

- *The fun network* is your support system for having a good time. These are people (perhaps people from your other networks) who are available for and enjoy the things you like to do. It is different from the friends network, in that your friends are yours, even if they are out of town, too ill to go anywhere, or busy. The fun network consists of people who are available when you are, especially if you work odd hours. If you're a parent, then other parents will want to do parent/child activities, like picnics in the park or going to see the latest children's film. If you're single, your fun network can help fill those times when people with families are unavailable, like weekends and the holidays. If you're married, the fun network can be others who will join you, with or without your husband, for fun times.

IDENTIFY INDIVIDUALS, TOO

As you can see, there are more than enough possibilities for support and networking. Once you connect with organizations and begin meeting people, you need to know how to identify the people who are most important to know, those who are most supportive and those from whom you can learn.

When you meet new people, keep in mind that your objective is to learn about them. As long as you observe the proper social conventions (dressing and behaving appropriately) you needn't worry about what people think of you. To worry about what other people are thinking is like getting inside their heads and looking through their eyes at yourself: it can't really be done—it's just a fantasy and will inhibit your real purpose, which is to observe them. Stay in your own head and concern yourself with observing what you can about the people you meet.

If you pay attention, people will usually tell you everything you want to know, without even being asked. You can interview new people without their knowing, and they'll feel complimented while you're doing it because you're giving them your undivided attention and interest. At a social function or private party, ask your host or hostess for an introduction to someone, or introduce yourself when he or she is not busy. Before you do this, have in mind something to say, such as, "This is a lovely party, isn't it?" Or, ask a specific question regarding something about the person. If you know his or her work, or have a friend in common, or even notice something interesting (like a great tie or gorgeous dress, great haircut, interesting pin or earrings), don't hesitate to let your new acquaintance know it. Everyone likes a compliment. In the appropriate social setting, most people, even the famous or well connected, will be friendly and willing to talk.

Often there are role models you would like to learn from or work with. Even famous people in your field, such as authors, are not always difficult to get to know.

> ***Robin*** *knew that the author of a book she admired lived in a nearby town. She did an Internet search, and was astonished to find the author's name and phone number. She called, fully expecting to get a secretary, but her author idol answered the phone! Robin recovered from her surprise and told the author how much she loved the book and asked if she could take a class from her. Within two weeks, she attended class and soon became the author's assistant. This famous author became Robin's mentor. "Am I glad I made that phone call," exclaims Robin now. "I never would have had all this help if I hadn't taken that chance."*

By selecting specific people you want to get to know, you can research them, find out about their work and interests, and prepare yourself for an initial conversation.

WORKING CAN BE PLAYING

Establishing a series of networks to make life and work easier helps you create a friendly, pleasant and helpful atmosphere wherever you are. You'll get as much gratification from giving help to others in your networks as you do from receiving their help. Working with people you admire and care about, laughing with friends and planning with colleagues can make work seem more like fun. No matter what you want to accomplish, or your chosen destination, friends and colleagues can make the journey fun. They'll be with you all the way, with support, companionship and information that you need when you need it.

9
Never Too Rich: Decide to Create Financial Security

***

A woman must have money and a room of her own.

—Virginia Woolf

***

To be secure and know that you'll meet your goals you need to know that you have financial health. No matter where you are on your road map, even at the beginning, if you manage your finances successfully you can create security for yourself. It's never too early to begin. No matter how small your income, you can begin saving and planning to invest. Although your mother and her mother may have depended on men (fathers, husbands) to make financial decisions, you should not be satisfied to allow someone else to be in charge of your financial future today.

WOMEN AND MONEY

A long time ago, through a local college, I offered an adult education class entitled "Women and Money," and a large group of women of all ages showed up. Some were young women, just out of high school or in college, who felt they needed to know about managing money and had never been taught anything about finances. Other women were a few years older, had children, and either were going back to work or getting divorced and wanted to understand and control their own financial affairs. Still others were much older, widowed and floundering while trying to manage the financial affairs they had previously let their husbands control. Most of these older women reported that they had gone from having their finances handled by their fathers to having them handled by their husbands. Some of the older women relied on grown sons to help them, but all of them felt that no one had ever informed them that they needed to be financially savvy. Even the educated women who were used to handling their own finances, found the more involved points about investing and planning for retirement and the children's education fairly overwhelming.

Traditionally, handling money was not considered "proper" for women, although financial surveys show that women often control most of the wealth in the world because men have shorter life spans and widows are left with the wealth the couple has accumulated during their marriage. Women are not the wealthiest people as individuals, but collectively we control more money and property. Because social mores have said that money and business are men's affairs, many women have become "money phobic" and either feel insecure about or unconsciously avoid money issues, sometimes leaving them in the hands of male accountants or relatives. "While nine out of ten women will be solely responsible for their finances at some point in their lives," writes Jennifer Parris, "few learned much if anything, about money and investing while they were growing up. And they regret it: 75 percent of adult women wish that someone had encouraged them or taught them about finances when they were young."

The very fact that most of the women in my class waited until after they were married (or even after their husbands had died) to consider the importance of being financially informed and capable demonstrates that these women did not think it was necessary for them to learn to manage money. While this is rapidly changing, and many women are completely comfortable and successful in financial dealings, this decision may be an important one for you.

> **Rita's** *father died when she was a teenager, and she watched her mother—who had been kept ignorant of financial matters—struggle to learn to write checks and manage money. Rita was determined to know everything about her family's finances, even though her husband earned all the money. As soon as she and her husband married (right after her high school graduation), she asked questions. As a result, Rita and her husband make all their family financial decisions together. When Rita was a full-time mom, the family finances left little room for saving, although her husband did invest in a retirement*

account at work. Now that Rita earns extra money, she contributes to a fund for the education of their children. She is taking an investment class and learning to invest in the stock market via the Internet. Her plan is to earn enough to put her children through college, and then to save for travel when she and her husband retire.

Every woman today needs to know how to manage her own finances. Rita waited until after she was married to begin to find out, and relied on her husband to teach her. While that worked for her, you can use the following information to begin to be financially informed now, whether you are married or not.

FINANCIAL ADVICE

While the days of face-to-face transactions with human bankers are being replaced by ATM machines and on-line investing, a banker should still be one of the first people in your financial network since it's his or her job to advise you in order to retain your business. Explore your local banks and savings and loan organizations, compare their features, and meet their managers. You've probably found the right bank when you find: a manager who takes the time to talk to you and explain what the bank has to offer for your financial situation; competitive interest rates; the services you want; and a convenient location. Banks sometimes offer free classes in investments and other financial topics. Your banker is also a good source for referrals to businesses and professionals in your area.

You may be eligible for a credit union through work, a professional association or other organization. Credit unions often offer the least expensive account fees, low-interest loans, automatic payroll savings deductions and excellent advice. In addition, they often offer special rates on car purchases, vacation packages and credit cards; and they like to educate their members.

A good certified public accountant (CPA) is another excellent resource who will help you avoid making costly mistakes. A CPA can easily save you more than he or she charges to do your taxes, will be there to help you if you are questioned or audited by the IRS, and can advise you on investments. If you are starting or running your own business, it is essential to have a good CPA working with you.

Financial advisors can also provide you with timely information to build your financial security. According to Oppenheimer Funds, Inc., it's important that you choose the person who's right for you. They advise that you: collect names from friends, family and colleagues; conduct interviews to find an advisor who listens to your goals and treats you with respect; check references and credentials; and keep your advisor informed of any changes in your financial situation. Search for How to Check Credentials on a Financial Advisor for several sites with good information.

If you're fortunate enough to have a financial advisor you already know, or one who is a member of the family, that is a great place to begin.

If you have a substantial amount to invest, or a lot of assets or property, take advantage of good advice but don't wait for someone else to handle your money. There are lots of classes, offered at banks, local colleges, and over the Internet, that can teach you investment strategies which will enhance the security of your financial arrangements.

Jodie took a crash course in finances. Her business was successful so early in her life that she had to learn about re-investment, profit and loss right away. Her advisor in Junior Achievers recommended a reliable CPA as soon as she began to be successful. When her business grew beyond her capacity to handle it all by herself, her CPA recommended a financial advisor, who counseled her about investing her profits and expanding the business. Now that she has begun offering franchises, she has been catapulted to a new economic level. Her financial advisor is putting her in contact with specialists in the franchising field who can help her set up her operation successfully. Her goal is to retire early. "I had to learn everything as I went along, and I had a tremendous amount of advice and help, or I could never have done it all," she says.

Kim was raised to be thrifty and concerned about saving. Her family had pooled all their finances to put her through school, and she was expected to succeed and help the next child in the extended family. Once she decided to be a pediatrician, she found a program that would pay for a lot of her medical school expenses in return for her promising to spend a few years working where they sent her. Because of this decision, and by living at home while she attended school, she was able to complete medical school debt free. She earned less than many M.D.s do for her first few years of working, but by living simply yet comfortably she was able to put some money aside. One of her cousins was a financial advisor and managed the family money. She trusted and followed his advice and carefully invested her funds, learning about stocks and mutual funds as time went by. She decided to invest half her savings in a deferred interest retirement account for herself and the other half in an account to be used for educating the next family member who showed promise. In this way, Kim took care of her obligations to her family and her own future.

Begin to Budget

Budgeting, like dieting, is one of those actions many women have good intentions about but don't seem to accomplish. The good news is that when you know how to do it, budgeting is much easier than dieting.

Step 1: Know Your Income

A good budget begins with knowing your personal financial picture.
Write down everything you earn. *If you get a salary, this is quite simple; just record your net pay. If you have several sources of money, such as child support, extra jobs, gifts from family or a small business, knowing your income can be more difficult. To find out what it is, you may have to keep track of all the*

money you receive by writing it down. There are several computer bookkeeping programs you can use. If your income varies from month to month, keep track of it for several months and then take an average (add together all your income for six months and divide by six to get an average per month).

Step 2: Know Your Expenses

Once you know how much money you take in, you need to know how you spend it. Keeping a record is the best way to do this.

1. **Write down your fixed bills.** *These include rent, utilities (gas, electricity, water, trash pickup), car payment, school fees (yours or your child's), insurance payments, real estate and income taxes (these are usually paid yearly, so divide by twelve), and loan payments. When you're done, you should have a list of all your fixed expenses—those bills you must pay every month.*

2. **Write down the rest of your expenses.** *These will vary with the time of year and the decisions you make about clothing, food, entertainment, self-care items like soap and toothpaste, etc. You will probably have a lot more flexibility in this category.*

3. **Analyze your expenses.** *One of the best ways to track fixed expenses is to pay everything by check or credit card and then analyze your checkbook or credit card statement after a*

couple of months. In these records, you'll have a listing of much of what you spent. If you spend much cash, write down all your cash expenditures for at least two months in a small notebook or expenses journal, or a phone app.

4. **Total your income and expenses by month.** *Then subtract the total expenses for each month from the total income for that month. Hopefully, you'll come up with more income than expenses, but for many women this figure turns out to be a negative number—which means they're sliding into debt more every month.*

Keeping track of your income and expenses, learning what you spend money on and how much of your income you spend, may be an eye-opener, but you'll find it is worthwhile to know where you stand. If you are earning more than you're spending, good for you! You can put aside some of the surplus for savings. If you're spending more than you're earning, you have to make some decisions. You can find ways to increase your income or you can spend less. Go back to your original list of expenses and see what you can leave out, or go back to your income and see whether there's any way you can increase it.

Once you know whether you're spending more than you're earning, or vice versa, you're ready to set up a budget.

Step 3: Set Up a Budget

Using your current spending as a guide, analyze what you are spending for each item: food, clothing, entertainment, transportation or auto expense, fixed expenditures such as rent, etc. Make a list of each category of expense and decide on an amount to spend each month on that item. Some people make this list on paper, while others use file cards or a computer.

> **Kisha** decided to cash her pay check, put 10 percent into savings, put enough into her checking account to pay her rent and utilities, and make an envelope for each other type of expense, such as entertainment, school expenses, groceries, and haircuts and clothing for herself and her children. She put the cash she had budgeted for the month for each expense into the proper envelope and would use the cash from the envelopes to pay for expenses in that category until the money was gone. If she didn't use all the money in the envelope that month, she let it accumulate. For example, if the children didn't need their school-expense money in the summer, by fall they had enough to go to the store and stock up on supplies just before school began. "Being a computer expert, I probably should have done it all on a computer program," she explains, "but I felt more in control of my money when I had the actual cash in my hand. It just worked better for me to use the dollar bills."

Budgeting can be valuable even if you're in better financial condition than Kisha was.

> **Jodie** had no money worries, but she quickly learned the importance of knowing how much she

was spending on each business expense, and it made sense to her to budget her personal expenses as well. With a good budget (or in business, a good financial forecast), she was able to plan ahead for improvements to her home and her business and to get the most out of her money. "Because I had a budget, when I wanted to help one of my cousins through school it was easy to know how much financial assistance I could offer her. Budgeting made me feel much more secure about my future."

How you decide to set up your budget (you may want to take a class, get instructions online, or get some advice from a CPA or a friend if the instructions above are not enough for you), plan how much of your income you'll spend on each expense, and stick to it. The point of budgeting is to live within your means and to provide for savings. No matter how much or little income you have, planning and using your money wisely will ultimately help you reach your goals.

SAVING MONEY

All financial security begins with knowing how to save. Kim and Kisha both serve as excellent examples of women who were able to save money with limited resources. Whatever your resources are, learning to plan and save money for financial goals as well as other career and life goals will make it much easier for you to succeed.

One of the most practical ways to save is to pay yourself first. Taking 10 percent or more of every dollar you earn and putting it aside *before* you spend money on anything else will keep you from going over your budget and guarantee that you create a financial base for investing. If you receive a salary, whenever you get an increase put the additional amount you get after taxes right into savings and continue to live on what you earned before. "Start by saving 10 percent of your income," suggests Henry S. Brock in *Your Complete Guide to Money Happiness.* "Join your company's investment plan (if you haven't already), or authorize a direct-deposit amount from your checking account into your savings account or a mutual fund every month." With regular ongoing deposits, your nest egg will increase fast.

Saving like this is a painless way to see your money grow and to be able to afford the house, the retirement investments and the vacations you have always wanted.

GETTING CREDIT

Your credit rating can be your biggest asset, but getting credit for the first time can be a bit of a problem—you must earn a credit rating; it does not happen automatically. If you were taught to pay cash for everything, you could be making a mistake by not creating a credit history for yourself. On the other hand, credit can tempt you to overspend and dig yourself into a financial hole.

To establish a credit rating, begin by using your phone or utility provider as a reference (if you've been paying those bills for at least a year) and get a credit card with a small limit (the usual starting limit for a first card is about $300). Make a few small purchases and pay them off right away to avoid finance charges, then watch the offers for other credit cards come in. Read the offers carefully, looking for the cards that charge no annual fee, offer benefits such as frequent flyer miles and have the lowest annual interest rates. Choose one or two cards and apply.

Credit cards are necessary if you want to rent a car, to buy something over the phone or the Internet, and for emergencies. You need one or two, but you also need to be careful not to overspend on them. Interest charges are exorbitant, so unless there is an emergency, do not accumulate a balance you can't pay off in the current month. If you want to buy something expensive, it's cheaper to finance it through your bank or credit union.

Though risky, credit cards can be used to keep track of certain tax-deductible expenses. If your CPA says your auto or travel expenses are deductible, for example, designate one card for auto repairs and gasoline and another for all your travel expenses. At tax time, the credit card statements will provide a record of all your deductible expenses. Remember, if you're using credit cards to keep track of expenses, you still must keep the charges within your budget allotments, and you must pay the account balance in full every month to avoid finance charges.

INVESTMENT OPPORTUNITIES

Although the vast number of ways you can invest and increase your money are far too widespread and change too rapidly to be adequately covered here, we will discuss a few of the most common ones. The best place to get specific advice for your individual situation is from your banker, CPA or investment counselor. Some of the most common ways for women to invest are real estate, the stock market, employer stock options, mutual funds, bonds, annuities, retirement plans and IRAs.

Real Estate

Real estate can be an ideal investment for women in most parts of the United States. You can decide to invest in real estate just to own your own home, which most investment counselors recommend, or you can invest in additional real estate as rentals, or to fix up and re-sell. Here, we'll be talking mostly about owning your own home or condominium. While it is true that real estate prices go up and down, and people sometimes lose their investment, it is also true that such people also have bought their property at a time when values are inflated, or refinanced a reasonably-priced property to the inflated value, so when the market fell back to normal levels, their loan balance was more than the value of the property.

Making decisions about whether the real estate you buy is worth the price, and will be a sound investment, is something to discuss with your real estate agent and banker or financial advisor. With careful planning, and good information about real estate prices in your area, it can be an excellent first investment.

__Kisha__ began with nothing and the extra expense of children to raise. As anyone with experience can tell you, making ends meet on welfare is not easy, but Kisha managed to save a bit. By working when she could and using her cooking talents to cater parties for friends, she made a *little money, which she used for extras, but she put 10 percent of it in savings before spending any. Her goal was to buy a condo to create a secure future for herself and her children. When she finished her computer-training program and began to earn a good wage, she put as much as she could aside, using the budgeting expertise she had from living on such a restricted income. She rented a four-bedroom house, which she shared with another single mom who had one child. This meant that their rent was a lot less than either would have paid alone, and they saved on groceries (by buying in quantity) and utilities, too. As soon as possible, Kisha invested in her company stock program and her retirement account. When she received year-end bonuses, she took a small amount out for Christmas presents and put the rest away. In a few years, she had saved enough for a down payment on a house. Her roommate had saved carefully, too, and since the two families had become very close, they decided to take advantage of a good buy on a duplex. They were on their way to financial security.*

If you decide that real estate investing is for you, ask your family, friends, associates or financial advisor to recommend a competent licensed real estate agent or broker. Talk with several agents until you find one who understands the kind of investment you want to make, whether you're buying your first home or investing in income property. A good agent or broker can refer you to reliable lenders, escrow companies, etc. advise you regarding zoning laws and the desirability of property location, and help you successfully negotiate your purchase.

> **Sharon** *had no financial worries, coming from a well-to-do family, but she knew that she still needed to know how to handle finances. Her family had given her money for college and helped her invest it and track the progress of her investment so that she created her own college fund from their initial gift. When her career opportunities looked limited, she investigated and found out that owning real estate was a very secure way to create income. She observed all the older people she could and discovered that the ones who were in the best financial shape owned rental properties. She took the remainder of her college fund, used it as a down payment and bought a fourplex in a modest neighborhood where property prices were somewhat depressed. She lived in one of the four units, renting out the others for enough income to pay the monthly mortgage and taxes. Because she lived rent-free, she saved a large portion of her salary for repairs and improvements to the building, plus future investments. After living in the fourplex for five years, she was able to afford a condo for herself in a much better area and eventually to buy more properties. Her plan is to pay off all mortgages in fifteen years and retire while living comfortably on the rental income.*

The Stock Market

When many women hear the word "investments," they think of the stock market first, which can seem fairly complicated and overwhelming. Investing in the stock market does require a lot of knowledge, and it can be risky, but there are many ways to learn. If you have the time and interest to really pay attention to your investments, you can do well in the stock market. Mutual funds and blue-chip stocks are more secure investments than you may think, and there are many courses you can take in investing to learn about them. The Internet provides both information and the means to do your own investing.

"If you're a novice investor," writes Nancy Gondo in *Investor's Business Daily*, "joining an investment club could be a great way to learn by doing, even with small initial amounts of money... The National Association of Investors Corp. (NAIC) (http://www.betterinvesting.org/) which offers educational products and start-up information to members, now has more than 37,000 clubs in its member base." Besides the booming number of clubs, there is an increasing number of women among club membership, as women have entered the business market, and want to learn about investing. The reputed success of many women's investment clubs may have also inspired women. When investing in the stock market, the NAIC encourages people to follow these four principles: invest a set amount regularly once a month, regardless of market conditions; re-invest dividends and capital gains; buy growth stocks; and diversify your portfolio.

If your employer is a big company (such as IBM, Xerox or Microsoft), it may offer an employee stock option plan, which allows you to invest a portion of your salary in corporate stock. Sometimes the employer will match your investment with company funds. If the company is secure, this is often the best way for an individual to invest. Many employees of growing companies such as Microsoft have become quite wealthy through their employee stock option plans.

Mutual Funds

Mutual funds are another investment option that is usually less risky than individual stocks. Mutual funds are a group of stocks put together by financial companies who hire experts to watch the market and design a portfolio of many stocks. You can buy shares in a mutual fund, and the seller will manage those shares for you. Mutual funds managers will provide you with information about their funds' investment histories and rates of growth. Your bank or your employer may also offer opportunities for you to invest in a mutual fund. Ray Martin, vice president of State Street Global Advisors, wrote in the *Bottom Line Personal* newsletter, that mutual funds are a wise investment choice if "you don't have the time... the interest... or the ability to pick stocks; you have only a few thousand dollars to invest and/or want to invest additional small amounts regularly, and... you want the benefits of diversification, but you don't have enough money to acquire a large portfolio."

If you haven't the time or interest to follow individual stocks or mutual funds closely, it will be worth your while to work with your financial counselor or buy stocks through a reputable broker who will advise you and will make a commission on each sale.

Annuities and Bonds

An annuity is a type of insurance policy in which you pay a premium now for a guaranteed income at retirement age. If you invest in an annuity, get good advice, because annuity quality varies a lot. Asking your financial advisor or taking a class in investing is often the best way to get informed about annuities.

As a teacher, **Marie** *had some special opportunities for investing. Federal law makes a certain type of annuity available only to teachers, and Marie invested everything she could in one. Meanwhile, she travels to Europe in the summers through education exchanges, teaching classes to pay her way, which keeps her from depleting her savings. This way she can enjoy her music and travel and prepare for her future, too.*

Many people invest in bonds, which are actually shares in government loans (a bond investor is loaning money to the government) initiated by governments to raise funds, and which are often tax-free and sometimes pay quite a dividend. Most of us are familiar with U.S. Government Savings Bonds, which are often bought as gifts for children, and which mature (attain their full value) in twenty years or so. While traditional savings bonds do not offer a very high interest rate, other kinds of bonds give you a much better return. Your financial advisor or bank can help you learn about investing in bonds.

Company Retirement Plans and IRAs

If you are employed, your company may offer a retirement plan in which you invest a portion of your salary and the company contributes to or matches it. These plans are usually only available to employees who've been with the company a number of years, and they vary in quality from excellent to poor. If you're fortunate enough to work for a company that provides a retirement account, ask a reputable financial counselor to look over the plan and advise you on the best ways to utilize its features.

If your employer matches some or all of your contributions, make every effort to contribute the maximum allowed. If your company offers stock options and is financially solid, stocks may also be a solid investment.

Even if you don't plan to stay at that company until retirement, you will benefit from the investment because you can withdraw your funds when you leave and reinvest them. Larger companies have personnel counselors whose job is to help you understand the retirement plan and other benefits, so take advantage of them if they are available.

***Megan** earns an excellent salary at her law firm and has taken full advantage of the opportunity to invest in its retirement account and have her contributions matched by the firm. She has resisted the temptation to spend her income on expensive cars, as her fellow lawyers do. She stays focused because she wants a family and she wants to be financially secure when she has* *children. She's taking care of her children before she has them.*

Traditionally, Individual Retirement Accounts (IRAs) have been and remain tax-deferred investments, meaning you can contribute a limited amount of money and not pay income taxes on it until you begin to use it at retirement (when you will probably have a lower tax rate because you have less income). The Roth IRA is taxable upon deposit, but the interest you earn is not taxable as long as you abide by the plan's rules. For the self-employed, several additional types of IRAs are available, with specialized rules. IRA funds can be invested in mutual funds, savings accounts, annuities, stock portfolios or other types of investments. Your financial advisor or banker can help you decide which of the many IRAs is right for you.

*With her early business success, **Jodie** needed some ways to minimize her income taxes, and her advisor recommended that she buy a house (to get the interest and maintenance deductions) and a Self-Employed Person's Individual Retirement Account (SEP-IRA) to allow her to defer some of her taxable income until retirement. "The whole financial investment field is very complicated," says Jodie, "and even with all my business know-how, I was overwhelmed by the possibilities. My financial advisor helped me sort it all out and saved me a lot of time. The investments are not only securing my future; they are also saving me a lot of tax dollars today."*

Making wise investments is one of the important ways to secure your future, and deciding to be financially secure means you will make careful choices about those investments. With help, and taking the time to learn what to do, you can plan your financial future quite effectively. Being financially secure gives you the solid base you need to realize the rest of your plans.

So far, all the decisions we have discussed are about how to make your life work the way you want it to, and to plan your goals and your road map for achieving them. The next chapter is about finding satisfaction and happiness along the way.

If you can do these things, you'll be focused enough that it will be easier to have fun. Good decision makers recognize that having fun is a way to recharge and energize and to enjoy life. Having fun enhances all your relationships; because when you're fun to be with, people want to be around you more. Remember, too, that women whose lives have a meaning beyond simply succeeding and accomplishing financial goals report more satisfying lives and relationships than women who do not.

10
Are We Having Fun Yet? Decide to Balance Work and Play

***

Each day, and the living of it, has to be a conscious creation in which discipline and order are relieved with some play and pure foolishness.

—May Sarton

***

The whole point of making good decisions early in life is to allow you to accomplish three things: to meet your goals successfully, to create a life that is meaningful and satisfying for you, and to be more efficient at the business of living to allow more time for fun.

THE VALUE OF PLAY

The value of work can be obvious, but what about the value of play? Recreation is aptly named, because it "recreates" or refreshes our energy and our motivation away from the seriousness of work and accomplishment. Play can be lighthearted and fun, but it is not meaningless: it is what we do so that we can work and achieve without burning out. While focusing on your goals and objectives, remember to balance your life with a proper amount of fun. "When you discard arrogance, complexity, and a few other things that get in the way," asserts Benjamin Hoff in *The Tao of Pooh*, "sooner or later you will discover that simple, childlike and mysterious secret... Life is Fun."

A generation ago, psychologist Abraham Maslow pointed out the importance satisfaction and fun played in the quality of life, with his concepts of the "self-actualized person" and of "peak experience." Since that time, research and philosophy has turned toward the search for happiness and meaning in life. In *Illuminata*, inspirational lecturer Marianne Williamson writes:

> *"The most positive breakthroughs of our times are internal. The drama of personal actualization is rarely reported in the popular press, except in irreverent, often ignorant, tones.... After centuries of looking to the outer world for our solace and power, we have begun to see the limits of a primarily external orientation.... We've embraced cold, technical, mechanistic reasoning (not that those are embraceable things) and suppressed our most essential strengths: passion, intuition, sense of the sacred, prophecy, vision and healing. And thus we have been controlled by thoughts, by*

institutions, by all manner of illusion.... Without our love, we're without our power.

"There's a consciousness we're capable of that integrates our various dimensions. It's joyful to be there because it feels like we've broken through constrictions which normally hold us back. This kind of spontaneous integration is not so out of the ordinary, so much as it is not part of ordinary conversation. It is under discussed and underinvestigated, invalidated as too soft or even ridiculed as nonsense. Although defined in psych ology as 'peak experience' and in physics as the 'flow,' this integrated consciousness is rarely appreciated for the opportunity it offers, to lead us up and out of our universal morass."

Because it removes us from our normal stressful environment, play has healing power. When you play, you are in a creative, spontaneous mode, focused on enjoying yourself and other people. In play, you are not focused on your problems or obligations but on what you enjoy. Making sure you have fun in your relationships and friendships keeps them strong. When we have fun together, we create good feelings that later become good memories. A playful mood can attract people to you because it's so attractive, and the contact that's begun there can grow into friendship.

Play can be overdone, of course: with too much focus on having fun, the essential obligations of life can be neglected. Although play is supposed to make people happy, playing to the extent that work is neglected does not make people happy and it creates problems.

Balance is the key: without fun, we lose our energy and pleasure in life, and it doesn't seem worth the effort it takes; without work, we don't accomplish what we want.

> *Jodie, with her business success so early in life, was at first thrilled to be so successful, and running her business was a lot of fun. After business had been her whole life for a few years, she began to burn out and resent the constant focus on work. She was short-tempered with her employees and exhausted all the time. Her decision-making ability was affected, and she finally sought help. She found a reputable therapist who helped her see that her business had taken over her whole life, and she needed a break. Jodie learned how to balance her time and to be sure she devoted some time to relaxation and play. She began to contact her old friends and make some new ones and resumed doing the things she loved to do. She found a friend to ride bicycles with, and she began going to movies and taking country western dance lessons. When she learned to balance work with play, her temperament improved, and so did her decision-making ability. "When I got away from work and responsibility for a while," she found, "I began to enjoy going in to work again. I wasn't tired of the company—I was just tired. Learning to pace myself better and take breaks made all the difference."*

The following guidelines will help you to balance work and play in your life:

Guidelines for Balancing Work and Play

1. **Set aside some regular time for play.** *Write it into your schedule and honor it as you would a business appointment.*

2. **Make a list of your favorite ways to play.** *Do you like movies? In-line skating? Singing? Dancing? Crossword puzzles? Playing cards? Internet Gaming? Sports? Spending time with friends? Think about all the things you can do and what feels like the most fun. List your favorites so when you want to do something fun you can refer to the list for inspiration. If you see or read about something that would be fun to do, add it to the list. When you have time, you will know what to do.*

3. **Utilize your fun network.** *Chapter 8 showed you how to create a fun network. Use it as a resource for people who want to have fun. Let them know you need to have more fun than you're used to, and ask them for suggestions. Learn from friends who are good at doing fun things.*

4. **Bring as much laughter into your life as possible.** *No matter what you are doing, if you add laughter it will become more fun. Don't be afraid to be silly or funny.*

5. **Leave room for spontaneity.** *Allow some time to do things on the spur of the moment. If you don't plan every moment and you allow yourself some free time, you'll find that spontaneous fun will begin to happen.*

6. **Do the sure things.** *If you know certain activities or people are guaranteed to be fun, do or see them periodically. If there's a movie that really makes you laugh, rent or buy it and play it when you need a boost.*

7. **Celebrate little things.** *Using the information you discovered in chapter 4, "Who Loves Ya, Baby?," about what constitutes a celebration for you, have a silly holiday. Celebrate getting out of bed on Monday morning, celebrate finishing a report and celebrate getting your car washed. Invite your friends for a picnic lunch, bring some cookies and soda to work, or have a virtual party with your on-line friends.*

8. **Find a way to recharge yourself spiritually.** *Try meditating, chanting, yoga, going to your favorite place of worship, communing with Nature, or attending a Twelve-Step group or a study course on the Bible, the Kabbalah, the I Ching, or A Course in Miracles.*

By planning to allow for fun and renewal in your everyday work plans, as well as on special occasions, you'll balance out your life and enjoy it more.

CELEBRATION

In chapter 4, we discussed the importance of celebration in creating motivation. Celebrating is a way to add fun to the challenges you face. If you know that each time you accomplish something you'll celebrate, your accomplishments will feel more significant and more worth doing. Most of us wait, however, until we've accomplished something really big before we feel it's okay to celebrate. Celebrating your wedding and your twenty-fifth anniversary, or even your yearly anniversaries, is not enough to balance out the hard work it takes to make a marriage successful; rather, it's important to celebrate all the accomplishments involved. To celebrate your graduation from college is truly wonderful, but what about celebrating each completed paper, each successful exam?

A change in your attitude can change how much fun you have. Instead of postponing your recognition of your accomplishments, learn to create satisfaction and fun by allowing yourself to celebrate small goals. If you have a successful relationship, you and your partner can tell each other every day how much you appreciate everything each of you contributes. Try having weekly "state of the union" discussions, during which you are sure to let each other know what you appreciate about each other, and watch your (and your partner's) satisfaction level in the relationship rise.

Ever since Norman Cousins wrote his books about healing himself through laughter, lots of research has confirmed that laughter and close relationships keep us healthy and make us live longer. "There's no question," maintains educator Sabina White of the Santa Barbara Laughter Project, "that laughter has both physiological and psychological benefits. Like exercise, it reduces tension... laughter gives the body a sort of mini workout. Like exercising, laughing involves virtually every major system of the body. Laughter is a cathartic, much like grief or anger... we all feel better when we laugh.... Why not laugh more and feel better?"

To have fun is to enjoy the results of your hard work and careful planning. A sense of humor can help you through the rough times of life, and laughter can change an argument into a reasonable exchange, or recharge and refresh you when you're tired.

Becoming aware of what makes you and the people close to you laugh can be a valuable tool for making your life and relationships work better. Notice what comedians you like, what movies, books, or humor writers amuse you, and learn from these clues to know what "funny" means to you.

SAVORING THE EXPERIENCE

Fun is not always laughter. "If you want to be happy for six months, get married," says a Chinese proverb. "If you want to be happy for the rest of your life, learn to garden." Marie knows that singing opera arias for an hour can restore her sense of inner peace and reduce her tension, while Robin runs every morning because it lifts her spirits and keeps depression away.

When Kisha was too poor to afford pricey entertainment, she 9 of us would call satisfaction. He found that:

"When you're in flow, you may be stretching yourself tremendously, but at the end you feel like you have relaxed physically. You may have been putting out a lot of effort, but you feel much more together and at ease than you have before.

"Flow requires investing all your attention in what you are doing. That acts as a kind of barrier against all the preoccupations that we have in life. If the relaxation has an activity look to it... that could be flow.... It means paying attention to what is happening around you so that you notice things, care about what happens, and forget yourself in the process. Whatever you are doing becomes very absorbing and interesting.

"When you get up in the morning, you try to figure out what about this day is going to be interesting or meaningful. You try to enjoy your breakfast, brushing your teeth, or whatever, you find a way to have an interesting conversation. That is what makes life worth living, not the things you will achieve tomorrow or the day after."

How do you "stay present" and achieve flow in your daily life? One basic method is to quiet your mind through meditation, quiet contemplation or prayer. Physical exercise with a spiritual focus, such as t'ai chi and yoga, are also helpful. But you can begin simply, just by spending some time in a place which makes you feel peaceful, whether that's a local park, your church sanctuary, or a special meditation corner in your room.

Surroundings of beauty can be nurturing to our most authentic selves, refreshing and uplifting us, as Thomas Moore eloquently describes in *Care of the Soul.*

> *"If we are going to care for the soul, and if we know that the soul is nurtured by beauty, then we will have to understand beauty more deeply and give it a more prominent place in life,"* states Moore. *"Religion has always understood the value of beauty, as we can see in churches and temples, which are never built for purely practical considerations, but always for the imagination. A tall steeple or a rose window are not designed to allow additional seating or better light for reading. They speak to the soul's need for beauty, for love the building itself as well as its use, for a special opportunity for sacred imagination. Couldn't we learn from our churches and temples, our kivas and mosques...? An appreciation of beauty is simply an openness to the power of things to stir the soul. If we can be affected by beauty, then soul is alive and well in us, because the soul's great talent is for being affected.... We don't often think of the capacity to be affected as strength, and as the work of a powerful muscle, and yet for the soul... this is its toughest work and its main role in our lives."*

SPIRITUAL VALUES

We hear a lot of discussion about values in the rhetoric of today's politicians and opportunists—to the extent that the word "values" has itself been devalued. However, the concept remains important to each of us individually.

It has long been known that those who live according to a belief system that carries a set of values and attaches meaning to their lives are happier and more satisfied with their lives, no matter what their economic status. As a modern woman, sometimes values and beliefs can be confusing, especially if your family espouses a belief with which you are not comfortable, or your spouse or children follow a different religion than you do.

But even if you and your friends, relatives or close colleagues have different philosophies, you will often find that the people you work, live and play with most smoothly have similar values, even if the ritual and traditions they use to express those values are different. As we discussed in chapter 8, your religion, Twelve-Step group or philosophical peers can form a social network that will support you in living by a set of values that gives your life meaning.

If you are fortunate enough to have been raised in a religion, a philosophy of life or a spiritual framework that gives you a sense of the value of your life and imparts meaning to your actions, all your decisions will be carried out within that framework. This is a great help, because, just as in having a road map, having a set of values you live by pre- determines many of your decisions. For example, if one of your values is to be honest and a situation arises at work where someone asks you to lie, your value system will guide that decision for you and your spiritual support system will back you up in telling the truth.

Spending time every day in prayer, meditation or spiritual study (for example, you study the Torah, pray, chant, "work a program," do transcendental meditation) will help you maintain your focus on your values and reinforce the meaning of your everyday actions. From prayer or meditation, you can recharge your spirit and refresh and reassure yourself that your life has value. Insight comes to us in these moments of opening up our awareness to the larger meaning of our lives. These insights can provide a whole new perspective on problems that may be troubling you and can give you new, creative ideas for accomplishing your goals, both spiritual and temporal.

All of us get tired and burnt out from time to time, feeling discouraged and lost. Having a spiritual resource, a philosophy or belief to turn to, can renew your energy and refresh your spirit. Your spiritual community, once established, will always be there to support, guide and comfort you in difficult times. In return, you can get great satisfaction from being there for others when they hit their low times.

Spiritual work can be tremendously rewarding, too. Volunteering in a program that has meaning for you, working with your spiritual group or support system, can be very rewarding. Tutoring, coaching sports or teaching art to disadvantaged children, leading a scout troop, feeding the homeless, teaching someone to read, visiting the aged or ill, or assisting at your child's school, pays no money, but the satisfaction you get provides a valuable return on your investment of time.

A support system based on spiritual values is a tremendous resource for increasing the level of satisfaction in your life. Such communities help us celebrate our accomplishments and support us in our losses and tough times. A spiritual community provides many opportunities to work together for what we collectively value and to give in a way that has extra meaning. Its value system becomes a guideline we can turn to when decisions become difficult.

Knowing that you are living your life according to what you believe, acting on your faith, and making decisions based on your value system all provide the kind of satisfaction that lasts, as opposed to more fleeting accomplishments, which will only provide short-term satisfaction.

Conclusion

The 10 Smartest Decisions a Woman Can Make Before 40 has given you the means for making practical, common-sense decisions. The more you become aware of the importance of your individual decisions, and the more practice you have at making them, the more automatic and easy they will become. Implementing them will give you the power to shape your life the way you want it to be. More important, you'll learn to be aware of the decisions you are making, whether you choose them actively or whether you make them by default, or by not making a decision at all. As you become aware of the power of your decisions and begin paying attention to them, you'll find that your decisions automatically become more thoughtful and carefully executed; and decision-making will be a tool you can use for your whole life.

Decisions are choices, and the power to make them is freedom. The ability to make good decisions means being in control and feeling confident and powerful. As a woman with more power than ever before, you have a greater need to know how to use it effectively. Because you can make decisions quickly and accurately, you can utilize your full power as a woman, a career person, a parent, a partner or a friend. In short, making good decisions gives you the freedom and the power to be your total self and to successfully meet the challenges life presents.

About the Author

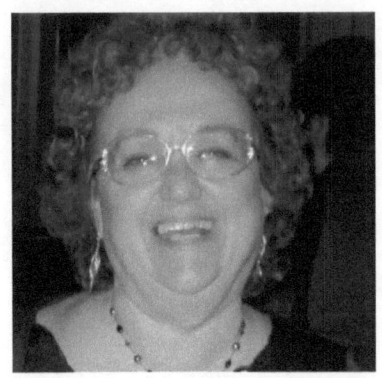

Tina B. Tessina, Ph.D., is a licensed psychotherapist in private practice in Long Beach, California, since 1978. She is the author of 15 books and has been published in 17 languages. Her practice includes individual and couple counseling, and she is a Diplomate of the American Psychotherapy Association and a Certified Domestic Violence Counselor.

Dr. Tessina's 40+ years of experience in helping people shows in her writing. Her books are very practical, filled with "reader-friendly" exercises, suggestions, guidelines, and examples. They are simply and elegantly written, yet powerful. Each book draws on the knowledge she has gained in her years of clinical work with individuals and couples, and was written as Dr. Tessina discovered a body of information needed by her clients. Her books are the result of her experiences in helping people improve their lives.

Dr. Tessina has appeared extensively on radio and TV, including To Tell the Truth, Larry King Live, Oprah, CNN, and ABC-TV News. She has written and been interviewed for Glamour, Marie Claire, Cosmopolitan, O, Time Online.com, and many other national publications. On the Internet, she is known as "Dr. Romance™."

In addition to her professional work, Dr. Tessina is a trained opera singer and a lyric coloratura. She also writes poetry and lyrics (her songs have been recorded by several well-known singers, including Helen Reddy), speaks Spanish and some French, and loves ballroom dancing. She lives in Long Beach, California with her husband of 36 years, Richard Sharrard, ballroom instructor and owner of DanceFactoryOnline.com. Tina and Richard enjoy traveling, their vintage California bungalow and their dogs.

Books by Tina B. Tessina

Dr. Romance's Guide to Finding Love Today
Https://tinyurl.com/y8tdwwje
*The 10 Smartest Decisions a Woman Can Make After
Forty* https://tinyurl.com/yctuql47
It Ends with You: Grow Up and Out of Dysfunction
http://tinyurl.com/z6xafbv
Love Styles: How To Celebrate Your Differences
http://tinyurl.com/h4xtnzx
*The Commuter Marriage: Keep Your Relationship
Close While You're Far Apart*
http://tinyurl.com/meaexzh
*Money, Sex and Kids: Stop Fighting about the Three
Things That Can Ruin Your Marriage*
http://tinyurl.com/l357zkl
*The Real 13th Step: Discovering Confidence, Self-
reliance, and Independence Beyond the Twelve-Step
Programs 3rd Edition* http://tinyurl.com/jlea2ru
*Gay Relationships: How to Find Them, How to
Improve Them, How to Make Them Last*
http://tinyurl.com/y9fqmnxw

With Riley K. Smith
How to Be Happy Partners: Working It out Together
http://tinyurl.com/zbe63u9
How to Be a Couple and Still Be Free 4th Edition
http://tinyurl.com/hbuhban

Browse these books at:
http://www.tinatessina.com/books3.html

Connect with Dr. Tessina online:

www.tinatessina.com
Twitter.com/tinatessina
Facebook.com/TinaTessina
Facebook.com/DrRomanceBlog

www.ingramcontent.com/pod-product-compliance
Lightning Source LLC
Chambersburg PA
CBHW051343280526
45784CB00007B/2796